AUSCULTATION OF THE HEART

WITH NOTES ON OBSERVATION AND PALPATION

RICHARD W. D. TURNER

O.B.E., M.A., M.D., F.R.C.P., F.R.C.P.E.

Reader in Medicine, University of Edinburgh
Physician and Physician in Charge of the Cardiac Department,
Western General Hospital, Edinburgh

FOURTH EDITION

CHURCHILL LIVINGSTONE
EDINBURGH, LONDON AND NEW YORK, 1972

CHURCHILL LIVINGSTONE
Medical Division of Longman Group Limited

Distributed in the United States of America by Longman Inc., 19 West 44th Street, New York, N.Y. 10036 and by associated companies, branches and representatives throughout the world.

© Longman Group Limited 1972

First edition	.	.	1963
Second edition	.	.	1964
Reprinted	.	.	1965
Third edition	.	.	1968
Fourth edition	.	.	1972
Reprinted	.	.	1974
Reprinted	.	.	1977

ISBN 0 443 00959 7

Printed in Great Britain by Butler & Tanner Ltd, Frome and London

PREFACE TO THE FOURTH EDITION

The suggestion that the text might be expanded into a book on Bedside Cardiology has in part been accepted by including notes on observation and palpation which may, in particular, facilitate diagnosis by auscultation. To produce a book on bedside cardiology would be a major task and change in policy, but certainly a stimulating exercise, and might prove useful.

I am most grateful to Frederic Jackson and Ronald Gold of Newcastle for helpful discussions, but they are not responsible for the final opinions expressed. I should also like to thank Anna Michelsen for remarkable patience in typing so many versions, and help with a comprehensive index.

1972   R.W.D.T.

PREFACE TO THE SECOND EDITION

This booklet consists of three articles written at the request of the editor of *Res Medica* in which journal they appeared in the summer and autumn of 1960 and the spring of 1961. They have been reproduced at the request of undergraduate and postgraduate students.

It is emphasised that auscultation can be mastered by all who will learn the underlying principles, acquire the necessary mental discipline, have the patience to listen to one thing at a time and seek every opportunity to practise. If what is heard is then carefully recorded an accurate diagnosis can be achieved in the majority of cases.

Since unnecessary anxiety is often engendered and unwarranted restrictions may be imposed as a result of misinterpretation, specialist advice should be sought whenever there is doubt as to the significance of the findings.

The rapid exhaustion of a first edition of 3000 copies within a few months reflects the need for a simple exposition such as this.

The opportunity has been taken to rearrange the text and to print the second edition in formal type with an improved cover. The author would be grateful for any suggestions as regards improving the text or diagrams.

I should like to thank Dr C. P. Lowther and Dr A. H. Kitchin for their practical advice.

1964   R.W.D.T.

CONTENTS

	Page
OBSERVATION AND PALPATION	1
AUSCULTATION	24
HEART SOUNDS	37
MURMURS	63
SUMMARIES OF COMMONEST DISORDERS	103
INDEX	119

OBSERVATION AND PALPATION

The introduction of laboratory investigations of many kinds has tended to be associated with less thorough bedside examination at which former generations were more practised. On the other hand the accuracy of certain observations has been increased by the introduction of special techniques which have also clarified the meaning of physical signs.

Some physicians are better observers than others and some take more care. 'Man sieht was man weiss', that is to say, the physician is more likely to detect disorders with which he is familiar.

OBSERVATION

Many general observations are relevant to heart disease and a remarkable amount of useful information may be gained by the use of the eyes alone. In the following paragraphs reference is mainly confined to observations which may assist the accurate and full interpretation of auscultatory findings of practical importance. Significant features include age, sex, anxiety, dyspnoea, pain, cough, hoarseness, flushing, pallor, cyanosis, jaundice, obesity, loss of weight, oedema and shock.

Particular attention should be paid to eyes, neck, hands and skin, to deformities such as sternal depression, kyphoscoliosis and spondylosis, and to general conditions such as pregnancy, hyperthyroidism, hypothyroidism, rheumatoid arthritis, scleroderma, gout, Cushing's syndrome, Marfan's syndrome and neuromuscular disorders. Alcoholism may be suspected from the face and demeanour.

Certain congenital disorders, such as Down's syndrome (mongolism), are frequently associated with heart disease.

Age and sex may be significant in that certain diseases more frequently occur in particular age groups and in one or other sex. The facies may suggest the diagnosis of at least an important associated condition almost at a glance.

Anxiety may cause circulatory disturbances including tachycardia, a raised jugular venous pressure and, of course, a variety of symptoms.

If the patient can be observed during an attack of pain it should usually be possible to determine the cause, and likewise that of dyspnoea which may take several forms including orthopnea, hyperpnoea, pulmonary oedema, Cheyne-Stokes respiration and hysterical hyperventilation.

Anaemia from whatever cause will aggravate symptoms and its correction may relieve cardiac failure or pain. Sometimes however it may be *due* to heart disease as in infective endocarditis or acute rheumatic fever. Severe, and especially acute, anaemia may be responsible for a hyperkinetic circulation.

Cough may be due to pulmonary oedema or related to pulmonary heart disease.

Cyanosis, if of central origin, limits the diagnostic field but if of peripheral origin usually reflects only a low cardiac output.

Jaundice may be due to pulmonary infarction, hepatic congestion from cardiac failure or, of course, a non-cardiac cause.

Pregnancy, owing to the increase in circulating blood volume, may be responsible for symptoms and signs which simulate heart disease or may aggravate heart disease.

Sweating may be due to anxiety (cold hands), hyperthyroidism (warm hands) or infection.

Shock may be of cardiac or non-cardiac origin and the cause must be determined.

Fever from any cause, and particularly when due to respiratory infection, may precipitate cardiac failure. Unexplained fever may be due to venous thrombosis or pulmonary infarction. If the cause of fever is not obvious in a patient who also has a murmur, infective endocarditis must be excluded as a first priority.

The classical mitral facies consists of high coloured cheeks with a blue tinge due to stagnation of blood in dilated subcutaneous venules and excessive extraction of oxygen. It is now less often seen and is characteristic of severe mitral disease especially if there is tricuspid regurgitation. It results from a low cardiac output and sluggish peripheral circulation usually with systemic venous hypertension. A similar appearance is rarely seen in patients with a low output from other causes, presumably because of the relatively short duration of their condition.

Examination of the eyes may show a premature arcus senilis or xanthelasma suggesting hypercholesterolaemia, petechial haemorrhages suggesting infective endocarditis, Argyll-Robertson pupils from syphilitic infection or Horner's syndrome.

The tongue may be pale from anaemia or show evidence of glossitis, but of greater diagnostic value is the blue discolouration of central cyanosis which is usually best recognised in this situation. Macroglossia may be due to amyloidosis which is one of the less common causes of myocardiopathy.

The heart may be involved in a variety of systemic diseases including rheumatoid arthritis, systemic sclerosis (scleroderma), disseminated lupus erythematosus, ankylosing spondylitis, neuro-muscular disorders and various less common conditions.

Skeletal deformities, as discussed below, may be responsible for apparent cardiac enlargement or be a factor in the aetiology of pulmonary disease.

Inspection and palpation of the neck, anterior chest wall and abdomen and examination of the hands will be discussed in detail.

PALPATION

Knowledge of the fact that there are at least fifty useful physical signs which may be detected by palpation in relation to the cardiovascular system should encourage the student to be methodical. With the advent of more elaborate techniques, clinical methods, including palpation, tend to be neglected and in consequence not only is important information often missed but unnecessary investigations may be carried out.

Bedside cardiology has the enormous advantages of availability, simplicity, safety and absence of pain and even discomfort. Confidence rather than anxiety is engendered by the personal touch.

In recent years instrumental methods, such as impulse cardio-graphy, have established the reliability of the information which can be obtained by simpler techniques.

Attention should be directed towards the chest wall, the neck, the abdomen and the peripheral pulses.

INSPECTION AND PALPATION OF THE NECK

The following points may be of particular importance under varying circumstances:

Distinction between jugular and carotid pulsations

Jugular venous pressure and pulse

Carotid pulsations

Carotid timing of cardiac events

Effects of carotid compression on heart rate

Carotid massage to terminate paroxysmal tachycardia

Carotid sinus hypersensitivity in cases of syncope

Carotid thrill

Kinking of carotid artery

Goitre

INSPECTION AND PALPATION OF THE NECK

Inspection and palpation of the neck should precede auscultation with particular reference to the jugular venous pressure and pulse and to carotid pulsation. In some cases the presence of a goitre is important.

Differentiation of carotid and venous pulsation

An inexperienced observer may find difficulty in distinguishing carotid from jugular pulsations, but with practice this is easily accomplished.

In the first place, an arterial pulsation is usually a single, brisk and palpable thrust, whereas a venous pulsation is more gentle and frequently has a double contour.

Palpation of the vessel is not always reliable because, occasionally, a vigorous presystolic venous wave may be easily felt.

Next, an arterial pulse is unaffected by respiration, posture or pressure over the abdomen whereas a venous pulse normally decreases with inspiration or sitting up and, conversely, is exaggerated with expiration, lying down and abdominal pressure.

Finally, if the *external* jugular vein is compressed in the supra-clavicular fossa the vein will fill from above, and can be emptied by compression higher in the neck with release of the compression lower down.

JUGULAR VENOUS PRESSURE AND PULSE

Close inspection of the jugular venous pressure and pulse may give very important information and sometimes the first lead to a correct diagnosis.

The examination should be made under optimal conditions with suitable and preferably indirect lighting, the patient comfortable and relaxed, reclining first at an angle of about 45° with the head supported and posture subsequently adjusted to give maximum pulsation.

Both sides of the neck should be examined because there may be differences. It is the deeply situated internal vein, which cannot be directly observed, that provides most information and acts as a convenient manometer of central (right atrial) venous pressure.

The characteristic 'welling' pulsation can readily be detected by the experienced observer but is frequently missed if attention is confined to the superficial external jugular veins. These veins are often obstructed as they pass through the fascial planes and are therefore an unreliable guide to venous pressure and pulsation.

The venous pressure may be considerably raised by anxiety, a fact which explains why this is sometimes evident at first examination in the consulting room or outpatient clinic, but not thereafter. The explanation lies in a redistribution of blood from vasoconstriction of the capacitance vessels.

In patients with heart disease, jugular venous pressure and pulsations are increased by exercise or even by raising the legs with the patient supine.

A raised jugular venous pressure reflecting right atrial pressure is due either to a rise in right ventricular diastolic pressure from cardiac failure, to decreased compliance of the ventricles, to tricuspid valvar disease or to cardiac tamponade.

Next, the effect of deep respiration should be observed. In health and in most patients with heart disease the venous pressure falls on inspiration due to increased negativity of intrathoracic pressure which facilitates venous return to the right atrium. By contrast, in expiration the pressure rises owing to increased positivity of intrapleural pressure which is transmitted to the cardiac chambers.

In patients with constrictive pericarditis or cardiac tamponade it may be noticed that there is a paradoxical rise in pressure on inspiration (Kussmaul's sign). This is due to the fact that the increased venous return cannot be accommodated.

Jugular pulsation

Normally two or three positive waves from retrograde transmission to the jugular veins may be observed with the individual lying almost flat. The first, or *a* wave, is due to right atrial systole and the second, or *v* wave, to right atrial filling with a consequent rise in pressure. A third, or *c* wave, shortly after *a* and coinciding with the first heart sound, is described by physiologists but is rarely visible in man and is probably usually due to closure of the tricuspid valve rather than to a transmitted carotid pulsation as previously thought.

The first negative wave after *a* is termed the *x* descent (systolic collapse) and is attributable to atrial relaxation and downward displacement of the tricuspid valve towards the apex of the right ventricle in systole.

The second negative wave, which follows *v*, is referred to as the *y* descent (diastolic collapse) and is due to the fall in right atrial pressure with opening of the tricuspid valve.

The abnormal wave due to tricuspid regurgitation is not an exaggeration of the normal *v* wave but occurs earlier in systole, and directly after or replacing the *x* descent. It should therefore not be described as a *v* wave, as is commonly done, but as an *s* (systolic) wave. Tricuspid regurgitation is probably present in most patients with severe cardiac failure.

In health presystolic *a* is usually the largest positive wave. An exaggerated or 'giant' *a* wave may be present if the right atrium contracts against resistance due either to tricuspid stenosis, a closed tricuspid valve as may occur in complete heart block, an increase in right ventricular diastolic pressure or decreased RV compliance due to hypertrophy from whatever cause.

In the presence of sinus rhythm the detection of a prominent presystolic wave may first lead to tricuspid stenosis being suspected and, if not observed, other signs may be unrecognised or misinterpreted. In this condition the *a* wave has a characteristic 'flicking' quality and may be so vigorous as to be mistaken for an arterial pulsation.

Regular, exaggerated or 'cannon' waves will be seen if the right atrium contracts against a closed tricuspid valve, as in nodal rhythm, or sometimes with 2:1 A-V block. For the same reason, irregular cannon waves may be seen in patients with complete heart block or extrasystoles. In paroxysmal ventricular tachycardia there may be irregular cannon waves from A-V dissociation.

In atrial fibrillation *a* waves will not of course be present.

In sinus tachycardia *a* waves may be fused with *v* waves.

In atrial flutter rapid, regular, small pulsations are frequently visible in the supraclavicular fossae.

With tricuspid regurgitation the normal systolic collapse or *x* descent following the *a* wave is replaced by a positive *s* wave. The tricuspid valve opens shortly after the peak of the *v* wave immediately following the second heart sound, and the y descent represents the phase of rapid, right ventricular filling from the atrium.

Numerous factors influence the y descent, including the height of the venous pressure, the pressure-volume characteristics of the right atrium and ventricle, and sometimes the presence of tricuspid stenosis. Prominent diastolic collapse is a feature of tricuspid regurgitation and may be the most striking abnormality to be observed in the jugular venous pulse.

In constrictive pericarditis there may be a sharp x descent but not a prominent systotic wave as in cardiac failure.

Carotid pulse

The carotid, rather than the radial pulse, is the best guide to timing of auscultatory events in the cardiac cycle. Exaggerated carotid pulsation is most frequently due to aortic regurgitation with a large left ventricular stroke volume. This was first reported by Corrigan who, incidentally, made no reference to the corresponding collapsing radial pulse as commonly thought.

Excessive pulsation may also result from coarctation of the aorta, in which case the femoral pulse will be weak and delayed after the radial.

In hypertension from other causes the pulsation is usually normal. Absent or unequal pulsations on the two sides usually result from atherosclerosis and this sign may be of value in the analysis of cerebral symptoms. Rarely it results from embolism or from obstruction due to a dissecting aneurysm of the aorta. In this context it may be noted that a carotid systolic thrill may have a similar significance.

In severe aortic stenosis the pulse is often of small volume and prolonged, but there may be little change until left ventricular failure supervenes. A pulse of normal volume may be due to some degree of associated aortic regurgitation which so frequently accompanies severe stenosis.

A double (bisferiens) pulse is often present with a combination of aortic stenosis and regurgitation.

Carotid compression may be used to slow the heart rate and thus facilitate timing in auscultation, to separate the two components of gallop rhythm, to terminate an attack of supraventricular tachycardia or temporarily change the degree of block in atrial flutter, or to confirm or exclude that hyper-sensitivity of the carotid sinus may be the cause of syncopal attacks or dizziness.

Carotid sinus pressure and massage

If light pressure over the carotid sinus does not influence the heart beat, firm massage up and down should be begun and maintained whilst counting mentally up to a maximum of about 10 seconds. A change of rhythm or cardiac arrest can be seen on the E.C.G., detected at the radial pulse or noted on auscultation.

There may be no effect, the paroxysm may be terminated, or the heart rate may be temporarily slowed. Cardiac arrest may occur and continue whilst pressure is maintained. If pressure is kept up for too long, syncope and convulsions may follow, but this of course should be avoided.

Correctly applied vagal stimulation by carotid sinus massage is often effective and the administration of drugs or electrical countershock rendered unnecessary. However, only paroxysmal atrial or AV junctional (nodal) tachycardia is likely to be arrested. There will be no effect on ventricular tachycardia but no harm results. In sinus tachycardia the rate may be temporarily slowed and in atrial flutter the degree of block is often transiently increased.

If massage alone is ineffective, administration of digitalis may bring about its effect. However, this drug should not be given if the use of electrical countershock is to be employed later, should carotid sinus massage fail. If massage does fail, and facilities for defibrillation are not available, the attack can often be terminated by the injection of a drug to stimulate the vagus.

Kinked carotid

A localised vigorous pulsation above the right clavicle may be due to kinking of the carotid artery from atherosclerosis, usually in association with a high aortic arch from unfolding. This condition may simulate an innominate aneurysm, which is relatively rare, but can usually be distinguished by palpation.

RADIAL PULSE

In the past, great emphasis was placed on palpation of the radial pulse but today, largely due to the corrective stimulus of direct arterial recordings, cardiac catheterisation and cardiac surgery, it has been realised that little reliable information can be obtained in this way, that is with sufficient precision to influence important decisions, such as whether a patient requires surgical treatment. This is because many factors influence the quality of the pulse.

The case of aortic valvar stenosis may be taken as an example. Relevant features include the degree of stenosis and of associated regurgitation, the calibre of the vessel, left ventricular stroke output, the cardiac output and the numerous factors which influence this, the peripheral and pulmonary vascular resistances and the presence of other valvar defects. Some of these factors are of course interrelated.

A slow-rising, sustained pulse of low volume is by no means always present in aortic stenosis but in fact is only found in advanced cases with a decreased cardiac output. The majority of patients requiring surgical treatment do not have the classical 'pulsus parvus et tardus'.

There may be some obvious abnormality, such as collapsing pulse, but in this case lesser degrees will more certainly be detected by palpating a larger vessel such as the carotid and, as regards an irregularity of rhythm, greater accuracy will usually be achieved by auscultation.

In particular torrential aortic regurgitation from the surgical point of view may be present without a collapsing pulse, and even without a full volume pulse if there is also aortic stenosis.

The correct interpretation of dysrhythmias and defects of conduction is greatly facilitated by correlation between palpation of the arterial pulse, auscultation, inspection of the jugular venous pulse and carotid sinus massage.

The radial pulse is often used to time events in the cardiac cycle, but greater precision can be obtained from the carotid pulse.

All this is not to suggest that palpation of the radial pulse should be abandoned because, not only does it establish initial contact with the patient and often instil confidence, but useful preliminary information may be obtained.

In the context of auscultation and the correlation of other physical signs, attention should be paid to rate, rhythm and quality of the pulse. Rates between 50 and 150 are usually physiological but these limits may be exceeded.

A rate greater than 160/minute, when not due to exertion, emotion or fever, is usually due to an ectopic pacemaker, that is to say, one outside the SA node, and attention should be paid to the jugular venous pulse, the heart sounds and the effect of carotid sinus massage as described above. A rate below 50/minute is usually due to heart block but may result from sinus brady-cardia.

The most frequent causes of an irregular pulse are sinus arrhythmia, extrasystoles and atrial fibrillation. Other causes include atrial flutter or atrial tachycardia with varying block and dropped beats from impaired conduction with the relatively slow pulse. A pulse of small volume reflects a low LV stroke volume and one of high volume is high LV stroke volume. Varying volume may be due to pulsus alternans or a varying duration of the preceding diastolic murmur.

Pulsus paradoxus

Pulsus paradoxus is a term in common use but a misnomer in that it reflects exaggeration of the normal respiratory variation in systolic pressure. In healthy persons this is rarely perceptible by palpation of the radial pulse, although systolic pressure may be decreased by 5 or even 10 mmHg with inspiration.

If suspected, confirmation should be sought by measuring the blood pressure. If the cuff is inflated until sounds can no longer be heard over the brachial artery and the pressure then allowed gradually to fall, it will first be noted that sounds are audible only in expiration. With a further fall in pressure, sounds will be heard throughout the respiratory cycle and, by convention, if the difference between the two readings exceeds 10 mmHg pulsus paradoxus is said to be present.

Pulsus paradoxus may result from rapid accumulation of a pericardial effusion, from constrictive pericarditis or from con-strictive myocardiopathy. It may, however, also result from any form of respiratory obstruction causing wide fluctuations of intrathoracic pressure.

Theories which have been proposed to explain pulsus paradoxus from cardiac compression include:

1. Dilatation of the pulmonary veins during inspiration with transient pooling of blood in the lungs and consequence reduction in atrial filling and in left ventricular stroke volume.

2. A rise in intrapericardial pressure during inspiration as a result of traction on the pericardium.

3. Competition between the two ventricles for a fixed total diastolic volume when the increased right ventricular filling on inspiration results in decreased left-sided filling.

Present opinion favours competition for space by the two ventricles in the distended pericardial sac as being the main factor.

Normally the inspiratory fall in *intra*thoracic pressure is equally applied to the left ventricle and pulmonary veins. There is no change in left ventricular effective filling pressure and no significant immediate change in filling or ejection. Right ventricular effective filling pressure does increase because the systemic veins are largely *extra*thoracic, thus increased filling of the right ventricle is without effect on the left ventricle.

When the pericardial sac is distended with fluid or constricted the effect is different. Increased filling of the right ventricle on inspiration increases intrapericardial pressure and hence impairs filling of the left ventricle.

Other signs of cardiac compression are described on p. 106.

Unequal pulsations

Unequal arterial pulsations are most often due to narrowing or obstruction from atherosclerosis but may also result from systemic embolism, congenital malformation or occasionally a dissecting aneurysm of the aorta. Surgical trauma, which includes cannulisation of arteries, is probably now the most frequent cause.

A particular example of unequal pulses is the subclavian 'Steal' syndrome in which narrowing or occlusion is responsible for vertebral arterial insufficiency with cerebral symptoms, sometimes aggravated by using the arm on that side. However, this interesting condition properly belongs to the domain of peripheral vascular disease.

In a patient with coarctation of the aorta, unequal pulses suggest that the obstruction is proximal to the left subclavian artery.

EXAMINATION OF THE HANDS

Whilst palpating the radial pulse for rate, rhythm and quality, the opportunity should be taken to examine the hands for features which may be relevant to heart disease.

Long, slender fingers (arachnodactyly) may be normal and sometimes occurs in families but also as part of the Marfan syndrome which includes cardiovascular manifestations such as dilatation of the aorta, aortic regurgitation, rupture of the aorta and various congenital cardiac anomalies.

Cold moist hands suggest anxiety, warm moist hands thyrotoxicosis and dry hands with a rough skin the possibility of hypothyroidism.

Unusually warm hands may be present with any high output state and cold hands with a low output.

Cyanosis is likely to be central in origin if the hands are warm, in which case it will also be obvious in the tongue. If the hands are cold and the tongue is pink cyanosis will be of peripheral origin, and the arterial oxygen saturation normal. Central cyanosis in a child and the association of central cyanosis with clubbing of the fingers is usually due to congenital heart disease.

Clubbing of the fingers in a patient with heart disease may be due to infective endocarditis, a right to left shunt or some associated but unrelated condition. Clubbing may also be a sign of postoperative infection, particularly after open heart surgery.

Anaemia may be obvious in the nails and if koilonychia is present iron deficiency is likely to be the cause. Whatever the cause, anaemia is harmful to those with heart disease and should be corrected. This may result, for example, in the relief of cardiac failure or of cardiac pain. Anaemia is usually present in infective endocarditis and acute rheumatic fever.

Splinter haemorrhages under the nails may be due to infective endocarditis but may be seen in otherwise healthy patients with valvar disease and are not uncommon in normal individuals, particularly manual workers.

Osler's nodes are painful, tender, reddish-brown areas in the pads of the fingers. They are uncommon but characteristic of infective endocarditis.

Rheumatic nodules are more commonly present over the occiput or elbows but may occur on the tendon sheaths in front of the wrists. In their presence active myocarditis can be presumed.

Rheumatoid nodules may suggest the cause of apparently idiopathic pericarditis. Systolic murmurs may also be present from involvement of the endocardium. Rheumatoid nodules may be present on the hands but more often near the elbows.

Gout is another form of arthritis which is occasionally associated with pericarditis. The feet should also be examined, and the hands for tophi.

There is probably a higher incidence of coronary disease in persons with hyperuricaemia.

Scleroderma (systemic sclerosis) may involve the fingers and be associated with myocardial fibrosis, pericarditis or, in advanced cases, cardiac failure.

Xanthomata may be observed as orange-yellow tinged streaks in the palms, as nodules over tendon sheaths or as raised eruptions in the skin. They suggest hyperlipidaemia which is often present with coronary atherosclerosis.

'*Liver palms*' may be due to cirrhosis of the liver in association with heart disease. However, palmar erythema is a non-specific sign.

Capillary pulsation, which is best seen in the nail beds after light pressure, is an unimportant sign of aortic regurgitation because, when present, there will always be more obvious manifestations and at an earlier stage. It may occur with peripheral vasodilatation with warm hands from any cause, such as a hot bath.

PALPATION OF THE ANTERIOR CHEST WALL

Apex beat
  Position
    Displacement of heart
    Cardiac enlargement
  Quality
    Left ventricular hypertrophy
    Left ventricular dilatation
    Double impulse
    Tapping impulse
    Triple rhythm
    Impalpable impulse
  Thrills
    Mitral regurgitation
    Mitral stenosis

Anterior ventricular wall
  Right ventricular hypertrophy
  Right ventricular dilatation
  Myocardial dysfunction
  Ventricular aneurysm
  Left atrial expansion
  Thrills
    Ventricular septal defect

Basal region
  Pulmonary hypertension
    Pulmonary arterial lift
    Pulmonary valve closure
  Thrills
    Aortic stenosis
    Pulmonary stenosis
    Patent ductus

Miscellaneous
  Dilatation of aorta
  Collateral vessels

PALPATION OF ANTERIOR CHEST WALL

Palpation should be carried out according to an accustomed regime, as with auscultation.

The patient should be supine and comfortably reclining on a bed or couch at an angle of about 30°. The observer should sit on the patient's right and apply the palmar surface of the right hand systematically to the region of the apical impulse, the sternum, the parasternal areas, the base of the heart and the epigastrium. A localised pulsation should be palpated with the finger tips.

After inspection of the chest to determine any abnormal contour or pulsation, the next step should be to determine the position of the apex beat. This is usually defined as the point lowest down and farthest out where the finger is distinctly lifted.

The impulse is normally within the left midclavicular line which usually in males corresponds to the nipple line, and in the fifth intercostal space, but is sometimes in the sixth and occasionally in the fourth space, depending on the position of the diaphragm.

The normal impulse consists of a brief outward movement at the onset of left ventricular ejection and is probably due to recoil of the heart against the resistance of the aorta.

An overacting impulse may be defined as one of normal form but large amplitude and may be found in healthy children and in patients with anxiety or hyperkinetic conditions, such as thyrotoxicosis.

If the position of maximal pulsation is outside the midclavicular line, in the absence of mediastinal displacement from skeletal, pulmonary or pleural causes cardiac enlargement can be diagnosed.

Common causes of displacement to the left are depression of the lower sternum and scoliosis, a fact which emphasises the importance of initial inspection.

Before deciding that the impulse is impalpable, dextrocardia should be excluded by palpation on the opposite side.

The impulse may be impalpable owing to obesity, a thick chest wall from muscular development, a rounded configuration of the chest which increases the distance between the heart and the ribs, emphysema, cardiac failure or constrictive pericarditis. Pericardial effusion does not usually obscure the impulse because, with the patient supine, the heart is displaced forward.

A sustained apical thrust is usually due to left ventricular hypertrophy (LVH). In dilatation of this chamber the pulsation is less forceful and more dynamic but hypertrophy and dilatation may be combined. However, there is often a contrast between the impulse in aortic stenosis from systolic overload and that in aortic or mirtral regurgitation due to diastolic overload.

A central thrust or lift in the sternal region, *best appreciated with the breath held in expiration,* is most often due to right ventricular hypertrophy (RVH) from systolic overload. It may also result from dilatation due to volume overload as from an atrial septal defect. It is often possible to distinguish these two causes but again there may be overlap. In particular, dilatation from increased volume load leads in time to hypertrophy.

A central lift may also be due to systolic expansion of the left atrium from mitral regurgitation. If there is gross dilatation of this chamber there may also be some pulsation to the right of the sternum and a rocking motion of the entire chest wall.

With enlargement of the RV, the heart may be rotated so that the apex is formed by this chamber, but in such cases there will also be a central lift. Likewise, with LV enlargement, this chamber may be responsible, not only for the apical impulse but for a central systolic lift between the apex and the sternum. However, LVH does not cause an isolated central thrust nor RVH an isolated apical one. With biventricular hypertrophy it is usually possible to distinguish two separate systolic thrusts of different qualities.

Palpation is a better guide to ventricular hypertrophy than electrocardiography because it is abnormal at an earlier stage. Radiography reflects cardiac enlargement but not hypertrophy, and considerable hypertrophy may be present without radiographic enlargement, as in isolated aortic stenosis.

An abnormal outward systolic pulsation to the left of the midsternal region may be felt after acute myocardial infarction or with left ventricular dysfunction during an attack of anginal pain, or from ventricular aneurysm.

A central pulsation is sometimes due to forward displacement of the heart by a pericardial effusion, hiatus hernia, eventration of the diaphragm or mediastinal tumour.

Occasionally the apical impulse is retractile during systole from constrictive pericarditis, tricuspid regurgitation or pleuro-pericardial adhesions.

A 'tapping' apical impulse corresponds to the loud first heart sound in mitral stenosis and is due to movement of the anterior cusp. It is not related to right ventricular hypertrophy.

Palpable pulmonary valve closure corresponds to a loud pulmonary component of the second sound and is due to pulmonary hypertension.

A third heart sound in early diastole, during the period of rapid ventricular filling, usually reflects ventricular failure.

A fourth heart sound in presystole is due to atrial contraction against resistance.

A pericardial 'knock' early in diastole is due to abrupt limitation of ventricular filling in constrictive pericarditis.

A double impulse on palpation may be due to subvalvar obstruction to ventricular outflow or to a palpable triple rhythm.

Thrills

A basal thrill usually arises from aortic or pulmonary stenosis, an apical systolic thrill from mitral regurgitation and an apical diastolic thrill from mitral stenosis. A left parasternal thrill is most frequently due to a ventricular septal defect.

Sometimes a diffuse systolic thrill with a 'purring' quality arises from rupture of a papillary muscle, and a continuous thrill to the left of the upper sternal border may be due to a patent ductus.

Occasionally a faint systolic thrill at the left sternal border is due solely to increased pulmonary blood flow, that is from an atrial septal defect, without pulmonary stenosis.

PALPATION OF THE ABDOMEN

Palpation of the abdomen should follow that of the chest, with particular reference to abnormalities relevant to the cardiovascular system.

Epigastric pulsation may be due to the aorta, right ventricle or liver.

With a hyperkinetic circulation from any cause, including nervousness, or even without this in a thin person, a normal aorta is often palpable. Dilatation of the abdominal aorta is usually due to atherosclerosis with or without aneurysm formation.

A palpable epigastric thrust from right ventricular hypertrophy usually also causes a lift over the lower sternum.

The liver may be enlarged from cardiac failure or cardiac cirrhosis. Systolic expansion of the liver is a characteristic finding in tricuspid regurgitation. In acute cardiac failure it is likely to be tender, and in cirrhosis it is firm or hard.

The spleen may be enlarged from infective endocarditis or cardiac failure but is often palpable in patients with rheumatic heart disease without these complications. It may also be enlarged in association with hepatic cirrhosis.

Systemic hypertension may be related to renal disease with enlargement of one or both kidneys.

Ascites in the present context suggests cardiac failure usually with cirrhosis of the liver or, less often, constrictive pericarditis in which case abdominal enlargement from ascites is frequently disproportionate to the relatively small amount of peripheral oedema.

The femoral pulses may be weak, or delayed after the radial, due to coarctation of the aorta. Either femoral pulse may be weak or impalpable from atherosclerosis, embolism or occasionally a dissecting aneurysm of the aorta.

EXAMINATION OF THE SKELETAL SYSTEM

Various deformities of the spine and chest wall may be significant in relation to heart disease. Important are sternal depression, scoliosis, severe kyphoscoliosis, and a 'straight back' (loss of normal kyphosis).

Scoliosis

Even a mild degree of scoliosis may be responsible for displacement of the apex beat to the left and hence a mistaken diagnosis of cardiac enlargement. This possibility should be suspected on examination from the front, with the individual standing, if the left shoulder and nipple are higher on the left side.

Sternal depression

Funnel- or cup-shaped depression of the sternum is rarely responsible for pulmonary or cardiac disorders but may lead to a mistaken diagnosis of cardiac enlargement from displacement of the apex beat to the left, or of valvar disease from the association of a systolic murmur.

Kyphoscoliosis

Deformities of the spine and thoracic cage may be due to congenital disorders, tuberculosis, rickets, poliomyelitis, muscular dystrophy and, less frequently now in most countries, empyema or surgical treatment for tuberculosis. When severe, these conditions may result in inadequate or uneven ventilation, compression of the lung, atelectasis, reduced compliance and a tendency to respiratory infections. The physiological and pathological consequences include arterial hypoxaemia, hypercapnia, pulmonary hypertension causing hypertrophy and dilatation of the right ventricle and finally cardiac failure (pulmonary heart disease).

Spondylosis

Spondylosis or spondylitis, involving the cervical or thoracic vertebrae, may be responsible for referred pain simulating that of coronary heart disease, as may any condition involving the same sensory pathways. Sometimes pain is felt also in the back, but nor infrequently only anteriorly. Pain may come on exertion ot spontaneously during the night or on the day following unusual exertion or posture. Thoracic kyphosis may also be responsible for referred pain which is aggravated by exertion. Skeletal pain is often relieved, at least partially, by nitroglycerin which, in consequence, is of little value as a therapeutic test in the differential diagnosis of pain in the chest.

Ankylosing spondylitis may be associated with aortic regurgitation.

Straight-back syndrome

Absence of the normal dorsal kyphosis, sometimes known as the 'straight-back syndrome', may be accompanied by a parasternal systolic murmur and unusually wide separation of the two components of the second heart sound. This murmur may be accentuated by external compression of the chest and decreases on deep inspiration.

Rounded configuration of the chest wall

A barrel-shaped chest may be due to an emphysema but is an unreliable sign. Emphysema may occur in its absence or may be severe with a normal-shaped chest. On the other hand, a rounded configuration of the chest wall may be responsible for relative faintness of heart sounds or murmurs owing to the increased distance and the tissues between the heart and stethoscope.

Neuromuscular disorders

There are a number of hereditary neuromuscular disorders associated with degenerative changes, fibrosis or hypertrophy of the myocardium. They are reflected clinically in enlargement of the heart, dysrhythmias, defects of conduction, triple rhythm, non-specific electrocardiographic abnormalities and cardiac failure. There is no specific treatment but the physician should be aware of the association of heart disease with, in particular, Friedreich's ataxia, pseudohypertrophic muscular dystrophy and myotonia atrophica.

The Marfan syndrome

The Marfan syndrome is an inherited defect of connective tissue and the clinical manifestations include skeletal and cardiovascular abnormalities and, particularly in the present context, dilatation of the thoracic aorta and aortic regurgitation. Other valvar defects and congenital lesions, and also dysrhythmias and defects of conduction, may occur.

The presenting skeletal features often include thinness, tallness, long slender extremities, arachnodactyly, deformities of the chest and spine, hyperextensible joints and deformities of the feet.

Dissecting aneurysm of the aorta may be a fatal complication.

AUSCULTATION

'I hear, I hear, with joy I hear'
—Wordsworth.

All students at first find difficulty with auscultation and to some heart sounds and murmurs remain a mystery. However, given sufficient interest, normal hearing, a good stethoscope and an appreciation of underlying mechanisms together with reasonable opportunity to practise, anyone can become sufficiently competent.

The essential requirements are a methodical approach with attention to detail and accurate recording of what is heard. This will usually lead to correct diagnosis.

Recognition of auscultatory phenomena is important, not only for accurate diagnosis but to avoid errors of interpretation and, in particular, the frequent error of suspecting or actually diagnosing heart disease when none is present and thereby engendering anxiety or imposing unwarranted restrictions. The latter may be a greater evil than failure to recognise mild organic disease.

The presence or absence of heart disease can frequently be determined by auscultation, but not the severity of a valvar defect nor, apart sometimes from the presence of triple rhythm, cardiac failure.

Undergraduates, of course, find difficulty from lack of experience and there is a danger that errors which are uncorrected at this stage will be perpetuated. However, difficulty is often largely due to lack of good technique and of appreciation that there is a rational and usually simple explanation for all that can be heard.

The adoption of a diagrammatic record of the auscultatory findings is recommended as a stimulus to accuracy, to save time, and to give an independent observer a clear idea of exactly what has been heard.

Postgraduate students are often more familiar with what they have been told or read than with bedside observation and tend to find physical signs which they consider 'ought' to be present rather than to record what can actually be heard. Objectivity is essential and the physician should record what has actually been detected and never what he thinks ought to have been heard, based on a preconceived idea of the diagnosis. Conversely, any findings which do not apparently 'fit' with the remaining examination must not be discarded without careful reappraisal.

Older physicians often find difficulty because they were trained before the days of modern precision which is due to the more accurate analysis of time intervals made possible by phonocardiographic studies, and the stimulus to accuracy provided by the information obtained at cardiac catheterisation or cardiac surgery.

Sometimes seemingly undue attention is given by specialists to what might be determined the minutiae of auscultation which may appear to be of academic interest rather than practical value, and at the bedside there may be a difference of opinion over detail even between practised observers. On the other hand, for example, the detection of a systolic click may signify that obstruction to ventricular outflow is at valvar level or, taken in conjunction with other evidence, closeness of an opening snap to the second heart sound will suggest that the degree of valvar obstruction is severe.

On occasion, phonocardiography is as indispensable to auscultation as is electrocardiography to the interpretation of arrhythmias, but most often it is used as a research technique to settle an argument or to provide a permanent record.

STETHOSCOPE

The practice of medicine is sufficiently complex without adding difficulties by inadequate equipment, and a small extra financial outlay will pay good dividends over the years.

Man mainly hears as he sees what he knows and the most important part of the hearing apparatus is the sophisticated computer which lies between the ear pieces of the stethoscope. However, it is surprising to find that some physicians, if few students, still possess a stethoscope with only a bell chest piece. Anyone having doubts as to the value of the diaphragm will soon have them removed by comparing the relative intensity of a high pitched murmur with both types of chest piece. The best example is the familiar early diastolic murmur of aortic regurgitation. Such a murmur is always better heard with a diaphragm and, if faint, may not be audible at all with a bell. Similarly, the low pitched, rumbling, diastolic apical murmur, which is characteristic of mitral stenosis, may be more readily heard with a bell and missed altogether with a diaphragm.

The modern stethoscope is a precision instrument which has been carefully designed to give the best acoustic performance. A popular and excellent model is the Littman stethoscope which has the advantages of being light and fitting conveniently into the pocket.

Transmission of sound is damped by air and consequently the length of tubing is important—the shorter the better. A length of 10 to 12 (25 to 30 cm) inches is suitable with an internal diameter of 1/8 inch (0.3 cm). Ear pieces should fit snugly so that the best size will vary between individuals. There must be no leaks from the system and good apposition of the chest piece with the patient's skin. The larger the area covered, especially by the bell, the better volume of sound obtained. However, if the bell is too large in a patient with a bony chest a complete seal round the edges will not be obtained without using moderate pressure. This may stretch the skin, thus converting it into a diaphragm and modifying what can be heard. In fact, varying the pressure which is applied by the chest piece to the skin is a useful measure of enhancing various sounds and murmurs, and full advantage should be taken of this. There is no mystery about these recommendations which are based on simple physical principles.

TECHNIQUE OF AUSCULTATION

Practice tends to make perfect, but everyone will agree that all the practice in the world will not necessarily make a good musician, golfer or physician. Nevertheless, skill with auscultation does come with practice and every beginner will be pleasantly surprised at how much can be heard when something has been pointed out and the lesson has been learned of *listening methodically to one thing at a time*. Auscultation should always be deliberate and never casual.

It is not necessary to be musically inclined to acquire skill in auscultation. A convenient simile is provided by the fact that, with practice in listening to a large orchestra, different instruments such as an oboe may be distinguished, whereas initially only an overall impression of sound will be appreciated. Likewise with auscultation, experience will bring appreciation of an added sound or high pitched murmur that has been missed by the relatively inexperienced or casual observer.

It is best to begin by concentrating on the normal heart sounds and trying to distinguish both components.

The mitral component of the first heart sound is best heard at the apex and the tricuspid component at the lower left sternal border.

The aortic component of the second sound is usually best heard to the right of the upper sternal border, or over it, and the pulmonary component to the left of the upper sternal border.

The component of the second heart sound that can be heard at the apex is usually derived from the aortic valve, the pulmonary component only being audible at the apex in cases of pulmonary hypertension or sometimes when wide splitting of the second heart sound, as in right bundle branch block, makes the separation of the two components very distinct.

After this it should be determined whether or not additional sounds are present and their positions in the cardiac cycle in relation to the two main sounds, preferably by indicating the interval in seconds after or before the nearest major heart sound.

Then, forgetting about sounds, attention should be paid to *murmurs*, first in systole, that is between the first and second heart sounds, and then in diastole, that is between the second and first sounds.

It is a good plan, having detected the presence of a murmur and its position of maximum intensity, gradually to 'edge' the stethoscope out in each direction to note its 'propagation' or 'conduction'. In some cases this procedure greatly facilitates diagnosis. For example, if a systolic murmur is loudest at the mid or left lower sternal border and can be traced best up and to the right, perhaps into the neck over the carotid artery, it is probably arising from the outflow tract of the left ventricle. If an apical systolic murmur is best conducted to the axilla, or beyond to the left lung base, it is more likely to be arising from the mitral valve and indicate mitral regurgitation.

In general, however, a murmur is also 'conducted' in proportion to its intensity and too much attention should not be paid to propagation.

Cardiac enlargement is another important factor. For example, with dilatation of the right ventricle, a tricuspid systolic murmur may well be heard at the apex.

The origin of the murmur may sometimes be determined by the accurate localisation of the corresponding thrill.

Full advantage should be taken of simple manoeuvres which may facilitate auscultation and hence accurate interpretation. These include posture, respiration, exercise, the Valsalva manoeuvre and occasionally the administration of an appropriate drug to increase or decrease systemic arterial resistance.

POSTURE AND RESPIRATION

Posture

In the reclining posture venous return to the heart is increased and this can be further augmented by raising the legs. Most murmurs and triple rhythms are louder in the lying position.

Mitral murmurs are best heard if the patient is turned on to the left side, bringing the apex of the heart closer to the chest wall. Mitral thrills are likewise best felt in this position.

An aortic diastolic murmur is best heard with the patient sitting up and leaning forward (with the breath held in expiration), advantage being taken of gravity.

If there is uncertainty as to the significance of a split second heart sound with the patient supine, auscultation should be carried out in the sitting position. If both components can still be clearly distinguished splitting is almost certainly abnormal (p. 45).

Presystolic and early diastolic triple rhythms are better heard with the patient supine, often when turned to the left side. Likewise, the associated additional impulse on palpation will be better appreciated in this position. Such added sounds and pulsations may disappear with the patient sitting or standing.

Respiration

Inspiration, by decreasing intrapleural pressure, increases venous return to the right cardiac chambers from the extrathoracic vessels with consequent prolongation of right ventricular (RV) systole and delay in pulmonary valve closure. At the same time, pulmonary capacity is increased with a resultant delay in venous return to the left atrium and consequent shortening of left ventricular (LV) systole and earlier closure of the aortic valve. As a result, right sided cardiac events are usually louder during inspiration and left sided events a few seconds later.

The effects of respiration are of particular value in regard to the two components of the second sound and to tricuspid murmurs.

Initially, auscultation should be carried out with the patient supine during quiet respiration, then, after instruction on how to breathe, whilst taking a long, slow breath, and then stopping *without* performing a Valsalva manoeuvre, and finally breathing out and holding the breath in full expiration.

In health, both components of the second sound can usually be distinguished at the end of deep inspiration, but fuse and appear single during expiration. If both components are heard in expiration it is probable that right bundle branch block, an atrial septal defect or RV dysfunction is present with prolongation of RV systole and delay in pulmonary valve closure (p. 45).

Occasionally the reverse obtains and separation of the two components appears during expiration owing to prolongation of *left* ventricular systole and delay in *aortic* valve closure. This 'paradoxical' splitting is a feature of left bundle branch block, severe aortic stenosis and LV dysfunction from coronary heart disease (p. 46).

The characteristic feature of an atrial septal defect is that the separation of the two components is 'fixed' and uninfluenced by respiration. This is because the pressures in the two atria are the same throughout the respiratory cycle owing to the communication between them (p. 46).

Right sided triple rhythms are usually best heard on inspiration and left sided triple rhythms on expiration.

Left heart murmurs are best heard in expiration, partly because there is less lung to dampen conduction between the heart and the chest wall and partly because blood flow through the left heart is greatest in expiration. Blood is held up in the lungs during inspiration, due to their expansion and the increased negative intrathoracic pressure. On the other hand, the intensity of right heart murmurs is often increased by inspiration when there is an increase in the degree of negative pressure in the thorax and consequently increased venous return to the right side of the heart. Under such circumstances the murmurs of tricuspid disease may be best or only heard. Tricuspid systolic and diastolic murmurs are frequently missed through failure to listen as a routine during deep inspiration.

When cardiac failure is present the heart may be maximally loaded even in expiration and consequently no inspiratory increase in the murmur is noted.

Exercise

Exercise is occasionally of value in bringing out a doubtful murmur, for example, a faint apical diastolic murmur from mitral stenosis by increasing blood flow. In the outpatient department the heart rate can be conveniently increased by 'running on the spot' with knees raised high, and in the ward by repeatedly sitting up to touch the toes and lying back.

Valsalva manoeuvre

In the Valsalva manoeuvre the subject is asked to carry out forced expiration against a closed glottis. This has the effect of decreasing venous return to the heart. On releasing the breath there is an *immediate* increase in right sided cardiac filling, which thus facilitates recognition of right sided events.

Drugs

The inhalation of amyl nitrite, which lowers the systemic vascular resistance, increases the intensity of left sided murmurs. Likewise, the administration of phenylephrine, which raises the systemic vascular resistance, has the opposite effect.

On occasion these may be useful beside tests when differentiation is difficult, but in practice they are rarely used.

AREAS OF AUSCULTATION

A word must be said about the 'conventional' areas of auscultation because, especially in patients with heart disease, they are often inaccurate, misleading and reflect outdated concepts.

The aortic area does *not* lie over the aortic valve and in any case an aortic systolic murmur is often loudest over the sternum, at the left sternal border or at the apex. An aortic diastolic murmur is *usually* loudest at the left sternal border. In aortic stenosis the pulmonary component of the second heart sound may alone be audible in the aortic area. In pulmonary stenosis the aortic component of the second sound may alone be audible in the pulmonary area.

In mitral disease the heart is usually enlarged and mitral murmurs or an important third heart sound are often loudest well to the left of the conventional mitral area. On the other hand, the mitral opening snap is often best heard close to the left sternal border. A systolic murmur due to mitral regurgitation from ruptured posterior chordae may be loudest in the aortic area. A systolic murmur, loudest in the mitral area, may derive from the tricuspid or aortic valves.

When the right heart is enlarged tricuspid murmurs may be heard best, or only heard, well to the left of the conventional tricuspid area and sometimes at the apex or in the epigastrium.

Errors of interpretation are not infrequently made through adherence to these conventional areas. It would be more accurate to use the terms aortic, pulmonary, left atrial, right atrial, left ventricular and right ventricular areas for the regions of the chest wall overlying these chambers. However, it is best to listen over the entire precordium, to describe the precise region in which sounds or murmurs can be heard and where they are loudest, and to draw conclusions from consideration of all the available data. Auscultation must to some extent be interpretative.

THE DISCIPLINE OF AUSCULTATION

'And sanctifying by such discipline
Both pain and fear—until we recognise
A grandeur in the beatings of the heart.'
—Wordsworth.

Sounds

Are both heart sounds present and, if so, is each normal?

If not, is the *first sound* louder or weaker than normal (or absent)? Can both components be identified?

Is the *second sound* louder or weaker than normal (or absent)? Does the second sound split normally on inspiration?

Is the splitting reversed, that is, widest on expiration?

Are there more than two heart sounds?

If so, is the *extra sound* in systole or in diastole? Is it nearer the first or the second sound? By what interval? What is its quality?

Is either sound preceded or followed by a murmur?

Murmurs

If a murmur is heard there should follow a similar mental catechism.

Over what area is it audible and where is it loudest?

In which direction is it next loudest or 'conducted', and how far from the position of maximum intensity can it be heard?

What are its time relationships to the heart sounds? Duration can be graded as short, medium and long.

Is it *systolic* or *diastolic*?

If systolic, does it occur in early, mid or late systole, or is it pansystolic?

If diastolic, is it early, that is immediately following the second sound, or 'mid', that is after an appreciable gap from the second sound, or late, that is presystolic?

As will become clear when dealing with individual defects and diseases, each of these features has a particular significance in diagnosis.

An attempt at grading the intensity and describing the qualities of a murmur should always be made. It does not matter how many grades are used by different observers so long as the standard is stated. This can be expressed as a fraction.

If, for example, a systolic murmur is recorded as grade 3/5 intensity, this signifies that the maximal number of grades recognised by the observer is 5, so that the faintest is grade 1, the loudest likely to be heard is grade 5 and the murmur in question is a moderately but not very loud one. An extra grade 6 should be reserved for the rare occasion when a murmur is so loud that it can be heard without placing the stethoscope on the chest wall.

As a matter of practical importance it is suggested that mitral systolic murmurs should be graded serially from the sternal border to the left lung base in order to facilitate comparison from time to time and especially before and after operation (e.g. 1234422). If intensity only at the apex is recorded an important change may be missed.

Grading by auscultation can only be approximate and variable because subjective. However, the three grades, faint, moderately loud and very loud, sometimes used are not sufficient if changes time to time are to be recorded.

As regards quality it would be helpful if agreement could be reached over adjectives, and preferably their number should be restricted.

It is suggested that the terms *blowing*, *harsh* or *rumbling*, and *high* or *low* pitched will cover most types or murmur. Additional terms are sometimes needed to describe unusual murmurs such as whistling, musical, raucous or the so-called 'seagull' murmur.

Murmurs often vary from day-to-day and hour-to-hour, depending on changes in cardiac output and blood flow. These in turn are influenced by rest, emotion, temperature, heart rate and other factors such as anaemia.

GENESIS OF HEART SOUNDS AND MURMURS

It is generally assumed that heart sounds are due to vibrations set up by abrupt changes in the velocity of the blood stream. Valve closure suddenly arrests or reverses the movement of blood and plays a major role in the genesis of normal heart sounds.

Until recently, murmurs were attributed to turbulence caused by excessive flow or by narrowing or irregularity of the channel through which blood is flowing. However, Bruns (1959) has produced evidence that murmurs are probably due to the creation of vortices in the wake of an obstruction or irregularity in much the same way as the Aeolian harp used by the ancients produced its tones.

This view lends credence to the observed fact of propagation of murmurs *downstream* from the valve producing them, as demonstrated by intracardiac phonocardiography and reflected in the different qualities of an aortic systolic murmur (p. 69).

From the clinical aspect sounds appear very short, but from the phonocardiographic point of view there is often no clear dividing line between sounds and murmurs.

In this clinical text the more familiar term turbulence is used, but with appreciation that it may not be strictly accurate.

PHONOCARDIOGRAPHY

Phonocardiography is the graphic registration of heart sounds and murmurs. A piezo-electric microphone is placed on the chest wall and the vibrations produced by the heart are picked up, amplified, filtered and recorded.

The crystal has the property of converting sounds or pressure waves into electric currents and responds fairly uniformly over the range of frequencies required in phonocardiography.

Phonocardiography has brought precision to auscultation and, having laid the basis for the correct appreciation of auscultatory findings, is now principally of use as a reference for accurate timing of events in cases of dispute, for teaching and research, and to provide a visual record, as may be necessary for publication.

Phonocardiography is no substitute for auscultation.

Heart sounds and murmurs are timed with an electrocardiogram. An external carotid arterial tracing, a jugular phlebogram or an apex displacement cardiogram or, on occasion, the pressure tracings from a cardiac catheter are also used as additional sources of reference. In some cases great precision has been obtained, particularly in children, by intracardiac phonocardiography using a phonocatheter which has the sound transducer at its tip. A more detailed analysis has also been obtained by some research workers using spectrophonocardiography whereby the grading of intensity and frequency of distribution can be recorded.

High quality phonocardiography demands good apparatus,

good technical assistance and, above all, the personal attention of a physician with plenty of time and patience and with knowledge of each patient and the points to be determined. In many cardiac departments these conditions do not obtain and hence recordings are of little value.

HEART SOUNDS

First heart sound   Mitral component
Tricuspid component

Second heart sound   Aortic component
Pulmonary component

Opening snap   Mitral
Tricuspid

Third heart sound   Right ventricular
Left ventricular

Fourth heart sound   Right atrial
Left atrial

Summation gallop

Ejection sound (click)   Aortic
Pulmonary
Mid-systolic

Pericardial sound (knock)

HEART SOUNDS

FIRST AND SECOND HEART SOUNDS

The conventional explanation for the *first heart sound* has been that it is mainly produced by closure of the mitral and tricuspid valves when ventricular pressure rises above that in the atria. In recent years this view has been challenged and evidence produced which suggests that the first sound actually follows valve closure and is due to vibrations in the closed cusps, chordae, papillary muscles and ventricular walls.

Likewise, the conventional explanation for the *second heart sound* has been that it is due to closure of the aortic and pulmonary valves when ventricular pressure falls below that in the great vessels. Again, recent work has suggested that the second sound actually follows valve closure and is due to vibrations in the closed cusps and adjacent structures.

Whatever the correct explanation, valve closure is the *determining* factor in timing.

Normally the sounds related to mitral and aortic valve closure are louder than those produced in relation to tricuspid and pulmonary valve closure because of greater pressures on the left side of the heart.

NOTE ON TERMINOLOGY

It has been customary to refer to the second heart sound heard in the conventional aortic area as A_2 and that heard in the pulmonary area as P_2 (p. 31). These are convenient abbreviations but, since the second sound consists of two components which it is important to distinguish, A_2 and P_2 should refer to the aortic and pulmonary components respectively regardless of where they are heard.

Heart sounds and murmurs may be difficult to hear on account of:

1. Thickness of the chest wall
2. Increased antero-posterior diameter of the chest
3. Decreased force of cardiac contraction
4. Emphysema
5. Pericardial effusion
6. Factors impairing conduction from the heart to the chest wall
7. Inappropriate stethoscope and chest piece
8. Impaired hearing, especially of high frequency murmurs.

QUALITIES OF THE HEART SOUNDS

The following properties should be noted:

1. Increased intensity
2. Decreased intensity or absence
3. Varying intensity.

Intensity of first heart sound

The conventional explanation has been that the intensity of the first sound in a normal subject is mainly dependent on the position of the valve leaflets at the onset of ventricular systole and on the force of ventricular contraction. More recently it has been claimed that the rate of rise of pressure in the left ventricle is the most important factor. Pathological changes causing thickening or rigidity are likely also to be important.

These assumptions will serve to explain varying intensity under different clinical conditions.

The first heart sound tends to be loud with *tachycardia* from any cause such as exercise, emotion, fever or anaemia and with other hyperkinetic circulatory states, such as thyrotoxicosis and pregnancy. The sounds tend to be faint in myocardial infarction or myocarditis, myocardial failure or myocardiopathy from any cause, mitral regurgitation and hypothyroidism.

If the valve is wide open and the cusps are far apart and have relatively a long way to go in order to shut, the closing sound might be relatively loud on this account, but if they are close together be relatively faint. The cusps will tend to be far apart if ventricular filling is prolonged, as from valvar stenosis or increased blood flow, or if the A-V conduction time is short.

In **mitral stenosis** the first sound is characteristically loud and slapping, providing the cusps are still mobile. This may in part be due to prolongation of atrial systole with the result that the valve leaflets are deep in the ventricle at the onset of systole, due partly to the shortened chordae tendineae holding the leaflets back and partly to the fact that the cusps are thickened as a result of rheumatic endocarditis. On the other hand, if the principal factor is a rapid rise of left ventricular pressure this could be explained by the increased left atrial pressure and some rigidity of the cusps impeding their movement towards the atrium.

In **mitral regurgitation** the leaflets may not come together at all, from structural defects or from widening of the valve ring, or they will do so imperfectly. Also, due to the double outlet for the left ventricle, the rate of rise of pressure in the ventricle is less. Consequently the first heart sound may be absent or weak.

The intensity of the first sound tends to bear an inverse ratio to the A-V conduction time as reflected in the P-R interval of the electrocardiogram, that is, the shorter the P-R interval the louder the sound.

Similarly, *variation in intensity* of the first sound will be present if there is dissociation between atrial and ventricular contraction such as may result from complete heart block, atrial fibrillation or flutter and ventricular tachycardia, when atria and ventricles beat at different rates. The varying intensity of the first heart sound in A-V block may be more related to different rates of rise of pressure in the left ventricle than to different positions of the valves at the beginning of systole.

The audible first heart sound is mainly related to mitral valve closure and it is rarely possible to distinguish changes in the intensity of the tricuspid component.

Intensity of the second heart sound

Normally in adults A_2 is louder than P_2 because the diastolic pressure in the aorta exceeds that in the pulmonary artery.

In children, P_2 may be as loud or louder because the pressure difference is not so great and the pulmonary artery is relatively large and nearer to the chest wall.

Either component may be loud, normal, diminished or absent, depending on intra-arterial pressure and valve movement, and on dilatation of the main vessel together with its proximity to the chest wall and its elasticity which facilitates valve closure.

Increased intensity of the second sound (S_2) at the base of the heart may be due to systemic or pulmonary hypertension. The relationship is not invariable and other factors influence intensity.

A_2 is by no means always loud even in severe systemic hypertension and loudness may be solely due to aortic atherosclerosis. In some cases of severe pulmonary hypertension from mitral stenosis, P_2 may not be loud, possibly from decreased blood flow. Thinness of the chest wall and dilatation of the pulmonary artery are other factors which may increase intensity.

Since pulmonary regurgitation is usually due to severe pulmonary hypertension with normal cusps, P_2 in such cases tends to be loud.

Decreased intensity or *absence* of A_2 or P_2 may result from deficient closure of the semilunar valves.

The *aortic component* may be weak or absent in aortic stenosis or regurgitation, and in such cases S_2 in the pulmonary area, which normally is finely split since closure of both valves can be heard here, will be single. If the *pulmonary component* is loud from pulmonary hypertension in such cases of aortic valvar disease it may also be heard to the right of the sternum.

The pulmonary component is usually weak or absent in pulmonary stenosis, so that S_2 may appear single and derives from the aortic component.

PHYSIOLOGICAL THIRD AND FOURTH HEART SOUNDS

A *third heart sound* may be audible early in diastole, that is shortly after the second sound and during the phase of rapid ventricular filling. It can often be heard in healthy young people.

A *fourth heart sound* late in diastole (presystole), that is just before the first sound, can usually be recorded by phonocardiography but is rarely audible.

These two extra sounds are described in the section on triple rhythm (p. 51).

SPLITTING OF THE FIRST HEART SOUND

The first heart sound is not a pure harmonic vibration but is composed of a number of unrelated frequencies. Normally four components can be recorded but only two are heard.

The first component may be due to atrial vibrations, as usually described, or be of muscular origin, as more recently suggested.

The second and third components are the principal ones and may be heard separately or as one sound and coincide with isometric contractions of the left and right ventricles respectively. These sounds are related to closure of the mitral and tricuspid valves.

The last or fourth component is probably due to systolic ejection of blood and may be vascular or valvar in origin.

Physiological splitting

Physiological splitting of the first sound results from slight asynchrony in ventricular contraction and is a normal phenomenon.

This can sometimes be appreciated in healthy subjects by listening at the lower end of the sternum, which is the position where the stethoscope is nearest to the relatively quiet tricuspid component, and by paying particular attention with the breath held in full expiration when there is relatively little lung tissue between the heart and chest wall.

The importance of a split first sound lies in its recognition and in differentiation from other conditions as described below.

Pathological splitting

Pathological splitting occurs in complete right bundle branch block when impaired conduction results in delay in right ventricular contraction and hence in loud splitting of the heart sounds.

DIFFERENTIAL DIAGNOSIS OF SPLIT FIRST SOUND

Atrial component of first heart sound

The atrial component of the first sound cannot usually be distinguished by ear but, in cases of partial heart block in which prolongation of the P-R interval of the electrocardiogram reflects delay in A-V conduction, this component may be heard and splitting of the first sound may be simulated.

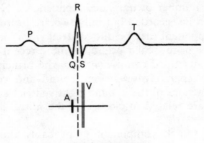

A = Atrial component
V = Ventricular component

Fig. 1 First heart sound.

Presystolic triple rhythm

Splitting of the first heart sound must also be distinguished from presystolic triple rhythm as discussed on p. 55 and from a first heart sound followed by an ejection click (p. 43).

In splitting, the two components are very close together and of somewhat similar quality. In presystolic triple rhythm, due to a fourth heart sound, the extra sound precedes the first sound by a wider distance and is softer and lower pitched in quality. An ejection click, on the other hand, is usually sharper and higher pitched than the first sound although it may be as loud or even louder.

Presystolic murmur

In mitral stenosis with sinus rhythm, atrial systole results in presystolic accentuation of the diastolic murmur at the apex. This murmur becomes louder when blood flow is increased by exercise or tachycardia from any cause. Most often such a murmur is associated with a loud first sound ('closing snap'), an 'opening snap' and a mitral diastolic murmur but, in patients with mild stenosis, only a short presystolic murmur may be present and in such cases there may be difficulty in differentation from splitting of the first heart sound.

Early systolic click or snap

Apparent splitting of the first heart sound may be due to the addition of an extra sound or 'click' which is sometimes termed the opening snap of a semilunar valve. It is synchronous with ventricular systole and in most cases probably arises from movement of the valve cusps. However, a click may also be heard with dilatation of the ascending aorta or main pulmonary artery and a normal valve.

It is often present in elderly patients and is then unimportant.

The added sound occurs soon (0.04 to 0.06 sec) after the first heart sound and is high pitched.

A click is of value in determining that obstruction to ventricular outflow is at valvar level. However, absence of a click may be due to rigidity of the cusps.

In patients with aortic stenosis or dilatation of the ascending

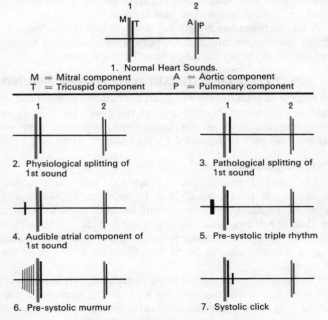

1. Normal Heart Sounds.

M = Mitral component   A = Aortic component
T = Tricuspid component   P = Pulmonary component

2. Physiological splitting of 1st sound

3. Pathological splitting of 1st sound

4. Audible atrial component of 1st sound

5. Pre-systolic triple rhythm

6. Pre-systolic murmur

7. Systolic click

Fig. 2 Differential diagnosis of split first sound.

aorta, this added sound is usually best heard at the left sternal border and sometimes at the apex.

In patients with pulmonary stenosis or dilatation of the pulmonary artery from any cause, including pulmonary hypertension, a similar sound may be heard and is usually loudest in the region of the second left intercostal space.

A pulmonary click differs from an aortic click in becoming quieter or absent with inspiration.

Differentiation from splitting of the first heart sound may well be difficult or impossible by ear and, without phonocardiography to determine precise timing, is largely dependent on associated circumstances.

Mid or late systolic clicks

Occasionally a systolic click is audible in mid or late systole, unassociated with heart disease. Presumably it arises outside the heart and probably from the pericardium.

A similar sound may also be heard in association with a late apical systolic murmur and has been shown to be due to unusual ballooning of the mitral cusps into the left atrium.

SPLITTING OF THE SECOND HEART SOUND

In routine examination of the heart particular attention should be paid to the second heart sound at the base. In difficult cases, when the diagnosis is not immediately obvious, very useful information may be obtained by attention to detail.

Physiological splitting

The normal second sound (S_2) has two components, as explained on p. 37, which can be referred to as A_2 and P_2 respectively, and every effort should be made to distinguish them by listening throughout the respiratory cycle. Usually the two components separate during inspiration and fuse on expiration so that if splitting can be heard on expiration it is almost always abnormal.

During inspiration the normally negative intrathoracic pressure becomes still more negative with resultant increase in venous return from the extrathoracic vessels to the right cardiac chambers. During deep inspiration this is exaggerated, stroke volume is increased, right ventricular systole is prolonged and pulmonary valve closure further delayed.

This is in contrast to the absence of any differential effect on *intra*thoracic structures which are equally affected by changes in pressure, so that the return of blood from the lungs to the left atrium is not similarly increased. In fact, expansion of the lungs results in a decrease in venous return to the *left* side of the heart and consequently left ventricular systole is shortened and aortic valve closure occurs slightly early. This combined movement of the two components of the second sound on inspiration results in their separation, often to a distance of about 0.04 second. When the increased venous return to the right side of the heart reaches the left ventricle there will be some delay in aortic valve closure, although to a lesser extent, owing to the dampening effect of the lungs, so that it is best for this test to be carried out after the breath has been held for a few seconds. After the breath has been held the patient should be asked to take a long, slow breath and then hold it *without straining* and then breathe out and hold it in expiration. The physician should listen during and immediately after each phase of respiration.

If separation of the two components is less than 0.03 second they cannot be distinguished and the sound will appear single.

Posture. The effects of posture on splitting of the second sound may be significant.

In normal children and young adults, expiratory splitting may sometimes be heard in recumbency but almost always disappears on sitting or standing up. However, if splitting is also present when sitting or standing, heart disease is likely to be present. In adults splitting which can be heard on expiration is always abnormal.

Pathological splitting

Abnormally wide splitting of the second heart sound is most often due to *delay in pulmonary valve closure* but sometimes results from *premature closure of the aortic valve*.

Delay in pulmonary valve closure may result from delayed activation of the RV or from prolongation of RV systole.

Activation of the RV is delayed in right bundle branch block, in which case the width of splitting increases slightly on inspiration.

Prolongation of RV systole may result from a relative increase in stroke volume compared with the left as in a left-to-right shunt through an atrial septal defect, from obstruction to RV outflow or from impairment of RV function. In such cases the degree of splitting cannot be further increased by deep inspiration and is described as being 'fixed'.

In summary, delay in pulmonary valve closure may result from delayed activation from right bundle branch block, from increased pulmonary blood flow, from obstruction to RV outflow or from RV failure.

Difficulty inevitably arises if one or other component of a split second sound is too faint to be heard with certainty or if it is obscured by a loud murmur.

Early aortic valve closure may result from decreased LV outflow into the aorta due to incompetence of the mitral valve or to a ventricular septal defect, when there is a 'double outlet' for the left ventricle.

Reversed (paradoxical) splitting

Prolongation of LV ejection or delay in its activation may cause A_2 to fall later than P_2, giving rise to audible splitting of the second sound on expiration. During inspiration P_2 moves in the usual way but *towards* A_2 instead of away from it, resulting in a single sound. This is the reverse of normal and hence the term reversed or paradoxical splitting. The most frequent causes are obstruction to LV outflow at valvar or subvalvar level, impaired myocardial function as from infarction, severe aortic regurgitation with an increased stroke volume and left bundle branch block.

Fixed splitting of second sound

The term *fixed splitting* of S_2 is used to describe failure of the two components to separate during inspiration. The classical example is in atrial septal defect. In this condition pulmonary valve closure is delayed due to the increased RV stroke volume which results from a left to right shunt giving rise to wide separation but, since the two atria are in free communication, they behave as one chamber, and the effect of inspiration is similar on the two sides of the heart.

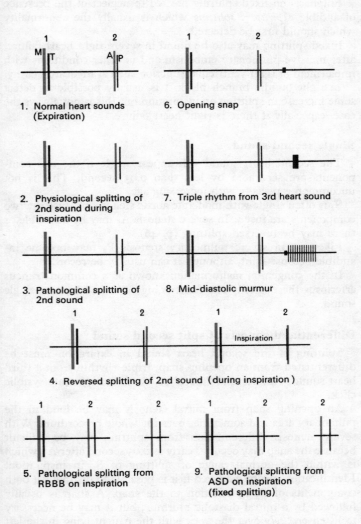

1. Normal heart sounds
   (Expiration)

2. Physiological splitting of
   2nd sound during
   inspiration

3. Pathological splitting of
   2nd sound

4. Reversed splitting of 2nd sound (during inspiration)

5. Pathological splitting from
   RBBB on inspiration

6. Opening snap

7. Triple rhythm from 3rd heart sound

8. Mid-diastolic murmur

9. Pathological splitting from
   ASD on inspiration
   (fixed splitting)

Fig. 3 Differential diagnosis of split second sound.

Emphasis on fixed splitting has led to neglect of the presence of audible *expiratory splitting* which is usually the abnormality which should first be detected.

Fixed splitting may also be found in severe right heart failure, after massive pulmonary embolism and in other conditions with impairment of right ventricular function such as myocardiopathy.

In right bundle branch block it is usually possible to detect some increase in splitting on inspiration but this is not always the case, especially if there is right heart failure.

Single second sound

The second heart sound will appear single if the two components are separated by less than 0.03 second. This is not uncommon especially with increasing age.

S_2 is often single with moderate aortic stenosis because the two components are fused. In severe stenosis A_2 may be inaudible or there may be reversed splitting (p. 46).

Likewise, in severe pulmonary stenosis P_2 may become inaudible because faint, although it can usually be recorded.

In the congenital malformation known as a common truncus arteriosus there is only one functioning valve and hence a single sound.

Differential diagnosis of split second sound

Splitting of the second heart sound in expiration must be differentiated from an opening snap, triple rhythm from a third heart sound, a pericardial 'knock' or, occasionally, a late systolic click.

An opening snap from mitral stenosis may be loud in the pulmonary area and sometimes over the whole precordium. With severe stenosis differentiation from splitting may be difficult because the snap may occur as early as 0.05 second after A_2, which is within the normal range of splitting of S_2 in inspiration. Identification can be achieved if it is possible to distinguish both components of S_2 in addition to the snap. A snap is usually followed by a mitral diastolic murmur, but it may be necessary to listen *precisely* over the apex with the patient lying in the left lateral position. A mitral diastolic murmur may be present without a preceding snap if the valve is sclerotic or calcified or if there is dominant regurgitation. Sometimes only a snap is audible after valvotomy.

If there is pulmonary hypertension P_2 may be fairly widely separated from A_2 as well as loud.

The interval between S_2 and a snap is usually between 0.06 and 0.10 second, and that between S_2 and a third sound between 0.12 and 0.16 second. A third heart sound can usually be distinguished from a delayed P_2 by its later occurrence, lower pitch and duller character. When associated with mitral regurgitation it may be immediately followed by a short decrescendo mitral diastolic murmur due to increased flow.

A pericardial 'knock' is usually sharp and the distance from the commencement of S_2 may be as short as 0.06 to 0.10 second. It may therefore simulate fixed splitting of S_2 or an opening snap.

Sometimes, of course, splitting of S_2 is present as well as one or other of these additional sounds. Differentiation is usually possible by taking all factors into consideration, including the finds on palpation.

TRIPLE RHYTHM

Third heart sound	Left ventricular
	Right ventricular
	Physiological
	Pathological
Fourth heart sound	Left ventricular
	Right ventricular
	Physiological
	Pathological
Opening snap	Mitral
	Tricuspid

Pericardial knock

Gallop rhythm

TRIPLE RHYTHM

*'This particularly rapid, unintelligible patter
Isn't generally heard and if it is it doesn't matter.'*
                                        W. S. Gilbert.—

So sang Gilbert fifty years ago, and so might some sing today with regard to triple rhythm, particularly perhaps physicians brought up before the days of modern analysis but not, let us hope, the student who has the opportunity to start aright.

Triple rhythm signifies that three heart sounds can be heard instead of the usual two, but this term should not be used to include splitting of the first or second heart sounds, that is to say, separation of their two components, nor for extracardiac sounds.

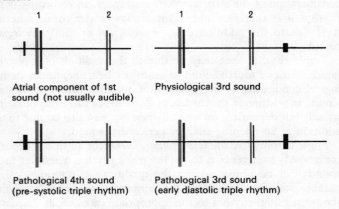

Atrial component of 1st
sound (not usually audible)

Physiological 3rd sound

Pathological 4th sound
(pre-systolic triple rhythm)

Pathological 3rd sound
(early diastolic triple rhythm)

Fig. 4 Triple rhythm.

An extra sound or 'click' which can sometimes be heard in systole, and is probably due to vibrations arising in a dilated pulmonary artery or aorta, is not usually included in the term (p. 43).

It is customary also to exclude the opening snap (p. 58). Certainly, this is an additional sound not normally heard in health, but it occurs only in mitral or tricuspid stenosis and is almost invariably followed by a diastolic murmur so that it is unlikely to be mistaken for any other sound and will be described separately.

All added sounds of true triple rhythm fall during diastole.

The terms third and fourth heart sound are, by convention, used respectively for the additional sound in early diastole due to rapid ventricular filling and that occurring in late diastole and dependent upon atrial systole.

Confusion over terminology from differences of opinion can easily be avoided by invariably qualifying the term 'triple rhythm' by its cause, such as triple rhythm from the addition of a physiological or pathological third heart sound, an opening snap or a pericardial 'knock'.

Triple rhythm may be physiological or accompany serious heart disease. Usually its significance can only be determined by consideration of the associated circumstances. In recording triple rhythm it is therefore important always to determine whether it is due to the addition of a *physiological* or of a *pathological* sound.

Triple rhythm then may be due to the addition of a physiological third or fourth sound in a healthy heart or, under pathological conditions, to the addition of an extra sound in diastole similar in position in the cardiac cycle to one of these physiological sounds but dependent on heart disease. It may also be due to the addition of an opening snap or pericardial sound.

Some authors use the term *gallop rhythm* for all third or fourth sounds. My preference is to use the triple rhythm whenever three sounds can be heard, adding the qualification physiological or pathological after considering the company it keeps, and confining the term gallop rhythm to the appropriate cadence, as discussed below (p. 57).

Not only has there been considerable confusion over terminology but great variability by clinicians in the recognition of triple rhythm. This is partly due to failure to listen with sufficient care.

The added sound in triple rhythm is usually of *low pitch* and occurs in a frequency range which it is relatively difficult for the human ear to appreciate. By the untrained observer these sounds must be specifically sought and it is necessary to listen intently and as specifically as does the trained ear which can pick out individual instruments in a large orchestra.

Triple rhythm is best heard with the patient supine and can be enhanced by raising the legs or by exercise, which increase venous return (p. 28).

Confusion has also partly been due to unawareness of the various conditions which may give rise to triple rhythm. It is not always appreciated that recognition is often rewarding not only by giving positive help to accurate diagnosis in disease and guidance on prognosis, but also as regards avoiding errors of interpretation, for example, of physiological sounds.

The detection of triple rhythm often provides the first clue to accurate diagnosis when the actual underlying condition has not hitherto been suspected. I have seen this in cases of myocardial infarction, constrictive pericarditis, myocarditis and myocardio-pathy.

It will be evident from what has been said that triple rhythm must be discussed as regards timing in the cardiac cycle and as regards its physiological or pathological significance.

By selective electronic amplification and graphic recording these sounds can be intensified and depicted for examination at leisure, as already pointed out, and in difficult cases phonocardio-graphy is an invaluable aid to precision in diagnosis. However, for most practical purposes, interpretation must be made at the bedside.

It is therefore necessary not only to be methodical in examination but to have in mind a clear terminology and classification.

EARLY DIASTOLIC TRIPLE RHYTHM

THIRD HEART SOUND

Triple rhythm from an added sound in early diastole, that is shortly after the second heart sound, may be due to a physiological third sound or to a pathological sound in the same position in the cardiac cycle and probably arising from essentially the same mechanism (Fig. 5).

It is best heard with the bell chest piece lightly applied to the chest wall and with the patient supine and turned towards the left or, better still, by direct auscultation with the ear applied to the chest wall, a practice which is too often neglected. It occurs between 0.12 and 0.16 second after aortic valve closure and is probably produced by vibrations occurring in the ventricles during the early period of rapid ventricular filling coinciding with the descending limb of the V wave (Y descent of the atrial pressure curve, Fig. 5). However, despite more than 50 years of experiment and discussion it is still not agreed whether this

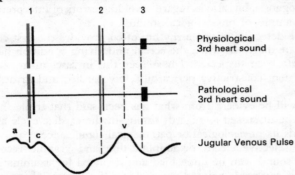

Fig. 5 Physiological third heart sound and pathological triple rhythm.

sound is of muscular origin from vibrations arising in the ventricular wall or whether it results from rebound tensing of the cusps and chordae of the respective AV valve on vigorous, early diastolic elongation of the ventricle during the rapid inflow phase. Whatever the mechanism, it corresponds with the period of rapid ventricular filling and, for this reason, tends to be loud when the ventricular filling pressure (atrial pressure) is raised and is never heard when significant mitral or tricuspid stenosis precludes rapid ventricular filling. The higher the left atrail pressure the earlier the AV valves open and therefore the earlier is the rapid inflow phase of diastole.

Owing to relative faintness and low frequency this sound can be recorded more often than it can be heard.

Physiological third heart sound

A physiological third heart sound is frequently audible in children and young adults but rarely in infancy and, for practical purposes, is so uncommon over the age of 40 that it should be considered pathological. The sound is accentuated by any hyperkinetic circulatory state, such as exercise, anaemia or pregnancy.

Pathological third heart sound

Pathological third heart sound, ventricular gallop and rapid filling gallop are terms sometimes used synonymously for one form of pathological triple rhythm which, as regards timing in the cardiac cycle and probable mechanism, is identical with its physiological counterpart, that is to say, at normal heart rates it is heard early in diastole and shortly after the second sound. It may be loudest at the apex or near the sternum, depending on which ventricle is involved, and also on other factors such as cardiac enlargement, rotation or displacement. A *left sided* third sound may result from systemic hypertension, myocardial infarction or any form of myocardiopathy causing left ventricular failure. It is commonly heard in severe mitral regurgitation.

A *right sided* third sound occurs frequently in massive pulmonary embolism and certain forms of cardiomyopathy, but rarely from tricuspid regurgitation.

The sound is of a dull, low frequency quality and is often

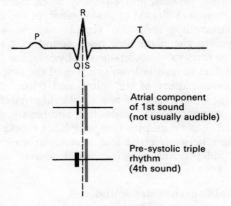

Fig. 6 Presystolic triple rhythm.

accompanied by a palpable impulse. It usually indicates **myo-cardial failure** from any cause.

Differential diagnosis is discussed on p. 60.

PRESYSTOLIC (ATRIAL) TRIPLE RHYTHM

FOURTH HEART SOUND

An added sound in presystole, usually referred to as the fourth heart sound, can frequently be recorded as a phonocardiographic event of low intensity and low frequency. It appears just after the beginning of the P wave and before the R wave of the electro-cardiogram and coincides with the '*a*' wave of the jugular venous pulse. It is probably due to a combination of vibrations produced by atrial contraction itself and vibrations set up within the ventricle as the consequence of the inflow of blood produced by atrial systole. Consequently it is lost with the development of atrial fibrillation.

Physiological fourth heart sound

The low-pitched vibrations which form the atrial component of the first heart sound cannot *usually* be distinguished in health. In a few normal persons, and especially when there is delay in A-V conduction (as reflected in prolongation of the P-R interval of the electrocardiogram), this sound may be audible im-mediately before the main first heart sound instead of being 'lost' in the louder, valvar component (physiological fourth heart sound). It differs in quality from splitting of the first sound (due to asynchronous closure of the mitral and tricuspid valves) in that the latter is composed of two similar high-pitched sounds. That atrial contraction can produce an audible sound is readily demonstrated in patients with complete heart block, when there is dissociation between atrial and ventricular contractions. In such cases independent, irregular atrial sounds can often be heard.

Pathological fourth heart sound

A distinct, presystolic triple rhythm is frequently heard in patients with **left sided heart disease,** particularly in those with left ventricular hypertrophy from *systemic hypertension* or following *myocardial infarction*. In patients with atypical features which might be due to myocardial infarction, it may give a useful diagnostic hint.

In many patients the clarity of this added sound and its distance from the first heart sound decreases with clinical improvement and in others, especially with systemic hypertension, there may be no change over many years without clinical deterioration. The sound, in fact, may be heard in patients with left ventricular hypertrophy from *symptomless* hypertension. Usually it reflects either left ventricular failure with a raised end diastolic pressure in the left ventricle or decreased compliance of the ventricular walls from hypertrophy. The sound may be *increased* by inspiration, exercise or elevation of the legs, all of which enhance venous return to the heart, or *decreased* by the Valsalva manoeuvre, sitting upright or venous occlusion tourniquets applied to the thighs which restricts venous return.

A pathological fourth sound is often inconstant and may, for example, appear during an attack of angina and disappear after its relief.

At other times, with worsening of the patient's condition and in particular with the onset of overt cardiac failure, a fourth sound may disappear to be replaced by a third sound, only to reappear with subsequent improvement and disappearance of the third sound.

Occasionally third and fourth sounds are both present, giving rise to a quadruple rhythm or, with tachycardia, will become superimposed giving rise to a 'gallop' (below).

In **right sided heart disease** a presystolic triple rhythm may occur from *pulmonary hypertension* or after massive *pulmonary embolism*.

GALLOP RHYTHM

When tachycardia is present the cadence of triple rhythm is often that described as a 'gallop', although not strictly comparable with the familiar sounds made by a galloping horse.

Because of its frequent association with myocardial failure this sound is often of serious prognostic significance and the louder the added sound the more serious the outlook.

A.O.T.H.—5

The term gallop should not be used as being synonymous with triple rhythm (p. 51).

Summation gallop

Summation gallop signifies the superimposition of atrial and ventricular added sounds. This may occur with prolongation of the A-V conduction time (P-R interval of the electrocardiogram) or, more frequently, with tachycardia.

Because of the loudness of this sound and its ready detection, summation gallop is probably the variety of pathological triple rhythm most frequently recognised and its association with tachycardia from ventricular failure is responsible for the gloomy prognosis so often associated with gallop rhythm.

Summation of the two added sounds can, of course, only be proved by the demonstration of quadruple rhythm with slowing of the heart beat. This can sometimes be achieved by pressure over the carotid sinus.

TRIPLE RHYTHM IN CONSTRICTIVE PERICARDITIS

A characteristic added sound early in diastole, somewhat similar in timing but usually a little earlier than other varieties of triple rhythm due to rapid ventricular filling, is often heard in constrictive pericarditis and may be accompanied by a palpable impulse. It is sometimes referred to as a pericardial 'knock'. It is associated with a prominent Y descent in the jugular venous pulse reflecting a high ventricular filling pressure. Doubtless both sound and impulse are due to a combination of rapid inflow from the elevated atrial pressure and the abrupt limitation of filling produced by the unyielding qualities of the fibrous or calcified pericardium.

Differential diagnosis is from a third heart sound and an opening snap (p. 60).

OPENING SNAP OF THE MITRAL VALVE

The opening snap of the mitral valve is a characteristic, high-pitched sound due to a sudden tensing of the anterior leaflet which is tethered like a sail at the mitral orifice. It is best heard with a diaphragm chest piece and is usually loudest between the apex beat and the left sternal border. It may be audible over a wide area of the chest wall.

In timing it occurs early in diastole (0.06 to 0.10 second) after the beginning of the second heart sound and shortly after the peak of the V wave of the jugular venous pulse, that is to say, immediately after the opening of the A-V valves (Fig. 7). If left atrial pressure is high, as is often the case in severe mitral stenosis, the valve will open sooner than otherwise. Consequently the interval between the aortic component of the second sound and the opening snap (2-OS) has been recommended as a guide to severity. However, taken in isolation, this is unreliable because factors other than the degree of stenosis also affect left atrial pressure, including left atrial volume and compliance, the cardiac output (which is itself influenced by a number of factors) and the presence or absence of mitral regurgitation. Nevertheless, when other factors are taken into consideration, it may be a useful additional point.

An opening snap can be heard in most patients with mitral stenosis of any degree whether or not this is complicated by regurgitation, provided that the anterior leaflet is still mobile. With heavily calcified or sclerotic, and hence immobile, cusps, the snap may be absent, muffled or soft. An opening snap is usually immediately followed by a mitral diastolic murmur. However, after a good mitral valvotomy sometimes only a snap may be audible.

In significance it has been claimed that a clear opening snap and loud first sound implies the presence of a 'pliant' or diaphragmatic valve with the inference that it would be readily amenable to surgical treatment. Although it does signify a mobile anterior cusp, experience has shown that it does not by any means follow that the adherent margins of the cusps will be easily separated and consequently that valvotomy will be successful. What the surgeon will be able to achieve cannot be predicted by auscultation.

Differential diagnosis is chiefly from wide splitting of the second heart sound, an early third heart sound and a pericardial knock (below).

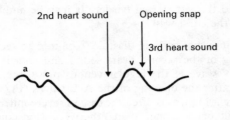

Fig. 7 Jugular venous pulse.

DIFFERENTIAL DIAGNOSIS OF THIRD HEART SOUND, PERICARDIAL KNOCK AND OPENING SNAP

A third heart sound, pericardial knock and opening snap each occurs as an extra sound early in diastole and may cause difficulty in differentiation unless all associated circumstances are taken into account. There is overlap in precise timing.

An opening snap from mitral stenosis usually occurs between 00.6 and 0.10 second after the second heart sound and is almost always followed by a mitral diastolic murmur. A diastolic murmur may not be audible if blood flow is greatly reduced by a high pulmonary vascular resistance, in which case there will be evidence of pulmonary hypertension (p. 105).

A pathological third sound usually occurs later than an opening snap (0.11 to 0.16 second) or pericardial knock, and is of a duller quality and may or may not be followed by a decrescendo diastolic murmur from increased blood flow. It is an important sign of severity in mitral regurgitation and may be associated with any form of myocardial failure, other signs of which should be sought.

A pericardial knock occurs slightly earlier in diastole than a third sound but more closely resembles a snap in quality, and is not associated with a murmur.

In all three conditions atrial fibrillation may be present.

Splitting of the first and second heart sounds is not included in the term triple rhythm because they are normal components of these sounds.

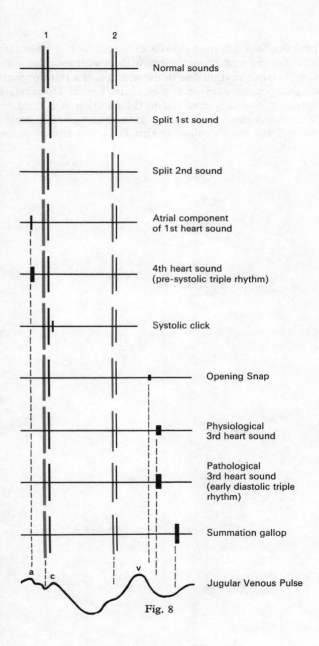

Fig. 8

Where doubt is felt over classification, clarity can be ensured by qualifying the term triple rhythm with an additional comment, for example triple rhythm due to the addition of a third or fourth sound, an opening snap or a pericardial knock. However, by convention it is usually confined to the addition of a third or a fourth sound. A third sound refers to the one occurring early in diastole and the fourth sound to that occurring late in diastole (presystolic).

MURMURS

The difference between a sound and a murmur is that the former is due to sudden alteration in the speed of blood flow whereas a murmur results from turbulence or vortices in the blood stream (p. 33).

A murmur is of longer duration and higher frequency than a sound. The principal factors which influence its quality are velocity of flow, density and viscosity of the blood, changes of calibre as regards blood flow through the heart, valves or large vessels, and irregularities of the endothelium.

It is remarkable that blood flow through the heart, round bends and past protuberances in valves should be so silent, and not surprising that minor irregularities of no structural consequence should sometimes cause eddies and be associated with a murmur. Another important factor is that a narrowed orifice, as from valvar stenosis, may give rise to conduction of a murmur behind as well as 'beyond' the obstruction.

A similar effect is produced by a relatively narrow vessel opening into a wider one, as in dilatation of the first part of the aorta or pulmonary artery.

Murmurs may be heard in systole or diastole or may be continuous throughout systole and diastole.

Diastolic murmurs are always due to organic disease and continuous murmurs usually so, but a systolic murmur is often present not only without functional disability but without any clinical, radiographic or electrocardiographic evidence of organic heart disease or obvious cause other than normal blood flow.

In all cases the area over which a murmur is heard should be noted and also the position of maximal intensity, the direction of apparent conduction, the intensity (graded), the quality (using simple adjectives) and, where possible, the precise timing in systole or diastole.

It should also be noted whether it is associated with a palpable thrill and if there is any abnormality of the heart sounds.

In cases of doubt, and when of clinical importance and not just a matter of curiosity, phonocardiography, radiography, electrocardiography and other accessory methods of examination may be required before a firm conclusion as to significance can be drawn.

Factors influencing the Character and Loudness of Murmurs

The qualities of a murmur depend on its spectrum of frequencies.

A low pitched diastolic murmur is usually due to low velocity flow through the mitral and tricuspid valves, whereas a high-pitched blowing systolic murmur, such as that from mitral regurgitation or a ventricular septal defect, is due to a relatively narrow jet of blood passing at high velocity from a high pressure to a low pressure chamber.

The chief factor influencing loudness is the rate of flow through the orifice or vessel responsible for the murmur.

Loudness will also depend to some extent on the proximity of the source of origin to the chest wall and on intervening lung which varies with the phases of respiration.

Changes in flow can be brought about physiologically by respiration or posture and by hyperkinetic states such as hyper-thyroidism, anaemia and pregnancy. Conversely, cardiac failure, pulmonary hypertension and hypothyroidism are conditions which reduce blood flow.

Variation in flow can also be achieved by use of the Valsalva manoeuvre and by drugs which influence vascular resistance, such as amyl nitrite or phenylephrine.

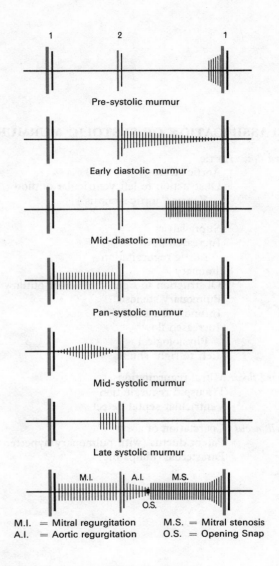

Fig. 9 Heart murmurs.

CLASSIFICATION OF SYSTOLIC MURMURS

Forward flow: Aortic
        Aortic sclerosis
        Obstruction to left ventricular outflow
         Valvar ('aortic stenosis')
        Subvalvar
        Supravalvar
        Increased flow
         Aortic regurgitation
      Pulmonary
        Obstruction to right ventricular outflow
        Pulmonary stenosis
        Infundibular stenosis
        Increased flow
         Physiological
        Left to right shunts

Backward flow: Mitral regurgitation
        Tricuspid regurgitation
        Ventricular septal defect

Miscellaneous: Coarctation of aorta
        Patent ductus (with pulmonary hypertension)
        Parasternal (idiopathic)

SYSTOLIC MURMURS

Systolic murmurs fall between the first and second heart sounds. They may occur in early, mid or late systole or occupy the whole of systole.

A systolic murmur may be due to various acquired or congenital defects or occur as an isolated finding unassociated with organic disease when they are sometimes termed innocent, incidental or functional (p. 80).

If a systolic murmur can be heard its characteristics should be noted, as described above, and also whether there is any accompanying thrill, diastolic murmur, change in heart sounds or other evidence of structural change.

In recent years the convention has been to divide systolic murmurs into two main categories of 'ejection' and 'regurgitant', the former being midsystolic or 'diamond shaped' on the phonocardiogram and due to aortic or pulmonary flow, and the latter being pansystolic, as in mitral regurgitation or a ventricular septal defect. However, there are a number of objections to this classification, which is essentially a phonocardiographic one (p. 81).

It is suggested that it is better to describe and record the characteristics which can be determined by auscultation in each case and interpret them in the light of all available bedside information and to avoid special terms, such as 'ejection', which has connotations that may not apply in the individual patient. However, a general classification is necessary and for this purpose the two main groups are due to forward flow, that is in the normal direction, and 'backward' flow, in an abnormal direction.

Aortic and pulmonary murmurs are due to forward flow from the ventricle through its semilunar valve. They occur during the period of ventricular contraction which begins with opening of the valve and ends with its closure, and consequently with the second heart sound and dicrotic notch of the carotid pulse.

At the bedside it is often *not* possible to hear both heart sounds and the murmur at the same time. Consequently, precise timing is impossible except by phonocardiography.

There is a short interval between the first sound and the onset of the murmur which corresponds with the phase of isometric contraction of the ventricle between closure of the AV valves and opening of the semilunar valves. Also the murmur may not necessarily begin with the onset of ejection of blood from the ventricle, in which case there is an interval before the velocity of flow reaches a sufficient level to produce a murmur. Some murmurs occupy only the mid-portion of systole but usually they continue with diminishing intensity up to the first, usually the aortic, component of the second sound. However, with severe obstruction to LV outflow and delay in aortic valve closure, there may be reversed splitting of the second sound (p. 46), and the aortic murmur may be heard beyond the pulmonary component. For similar reasons the murmur of pulmonary valve stenosis may extend beyond the aortic component to end with the pulmonary component of the second sound which may be delayed by prolongation of RV systole.

Likewise, with backward flow due to mitral or tricuspid regurgitation or to a ventricular septal defect, a murmur is often audible throughout the period when a gradient is present, but various factors may modify this situation in individual cases so that again generalisations do not necessarily apply. Such murmurs are by no means always pansystolic.

These facts need not confuse the beginner and are mentioned to stimulate interest and to illustrate principles. In practice, when surgical treatment is under consideration the precise nature and severity of a structural defect must be determined by considering all available information. Sometimes this must include special laboratory investigations. Often, however, accurate interpretation by physical signs will suffice.

BASAL SYSTOLIC MURMURS

Basal systolic murmurs most often derive from the aortic or pulmonary valve. Sometimes they are transmitted from elsewhere, for example, mitral regurgitation with a jet directed upwards rather than backwards.

AORTIC SYSTOLIC MURMURS

The most frequent cause for a systolic murmur, which is loudest in the true aortic area (p. 30), is obstruction to left ventricular outflow at the valve. Less commonly obstruction is below, and rarely above, the valve.

A similar murmur may be due to valvar sclerosis without stenosis, to relative stenosis from dilatation of the ascending aorta or to increased left ventricular stroke volume.

Aortic valvar stenosis

Characteristically the murmur of aortic valvar stenosis is harsh and loudest in midsystole because this corresponds to the period of maximal blood flow. On the phonocardiogram the configuration is often that of a diamond (Fig. 9). An aortic systolic murmur may be loudest to the right of the upper sternal border, over the sternum, down the left sternal border or sometimes even at the apex. Often, but by no means always, it is audible over the carotid arteries. Even when the murmur is not loudest to the right of the upper sternum, its origin may be recognised because it is also audible in this region and has similar timing.

The *quality* of the murmur is often more musical towards the apex, a dissociation which was first noticed by Gallavardin.

If the cusps are sclerotic or calcified, A_2 may be faint or absent. If only P_2 can be heard, it may be possible to appreciate by ear that the murmur ends before it. Sometimes also it can be appreciated that there is a distinct gap between the first heart sound and the beginning of the murmur. However, in many cases one or other or both heart sounds cannot be heard, making precise timing impossible except by phonocardiography when simultaneous recordings can be recorded from several areas. Also the position in systole of maximal intensity depends on the degree of obstruction, being later with severe stenosis. These are some of the reasons for avoiding the term 'ejection' (p. 81).

It is important to emphasise that the loudness of the murmur bears no close relationship to the degree of obstruction. In fact intensity is usually greatest with moderate stenosis. In severe cases, especially if there is left ventricular failure, the murmur may be faint or disappear.

There may or may not be an accompanying thrill but the intensity of the murmur does not always correspond to that of the thrill. Occasionally, even with a harsh murmur and thrill, there is no pressure gradient across the valve.

If the cusps are rigid and immobile there is usually an early diastolic murmur from associated aortic regurgitation.

The causes of aortic valvar stenosis are rheumatic fever, a congenital dome-shaped deformity or a congenital bicuspid valve with sclerosis or calcification.

Subvalvar stenosis obstruction to left ventricular outflow is sometimes at subvalvar level. This may be due to muscular hypertrophy of the septum (myocardiopathy) or occasionally to a fibrous diaphragm.

Supravalvar stenosis to outflow in various forms may also occur as a congenital malformation of the ascending aorta.

These conditions should be suspected if there are atypical features for valvar stenosis, such as absence of calcification, the presence of an ejection click or if the murmur and thrill are lower or higher in position than is usual for valvar stenosis.

Sclerosis of the cusps without significant stenosis is a common cause for an aortic systolic murmur in the elderly, especially in males.

A similar murmur may be found in apparently healthy young persons from a congenitally malformed and usually bicuspid valve. In a proportion (unknown) of such cases, progressive sclerosis or calcification is responsible for severe valvar stenosis in later life.

Increased blood flow from a large stroke output, as in aortic regurgitation, may also be responsible for a systolic murmur and be present without any gradient across the valve.

Dilatation of the first part of the aorta with consequent relative stenosis of the valve may likewise result in sufficient turbulence to produce a murmur.

Isolated supraclavicular systolic murmur

A systolic murmur above the clavicles may be due to carotid or subclavian arterial stenosis. However, it is important to know that a similar murmur is frequently audible in health, especially in the young, and occasionally in such cases may also be heard just below the clavicle and hence be mistaken for valvar disease. It probably arises from the impingement of blood on the bifurcation of the innominate artery or possibly derive from the subclavian artery.

DIFFERENTIAL DIAGNOSIS

If the classical clinical features are present, a systolic murmur, maximal in the *conventional* aortic area, is most often due to aortic valvar stenosis but, as discussed above, there are other causes for such a murmur. Also an aortic systolic murmur may be audible anywhere over the *true* aortic area or at the apex.

An associated aortic diastolic murmur favours valvar stenosis as does an opening snap (ejection click). If calcification of the valve can be seen on radioscopy the valvar origin of the murmur can be assumed but, if not present, then other possible causes should be carefully considered.

Dilatation of the ascending aorta also favours valvar stenosis.

It bears repetition that an aortic systolic murmur is *not* always loudest in the conventional aortic area or conducted into the carotids, its intensity bears *no* close relation to the severity of the underlying structural defect and it is *not* always accompanied by a thrill.

If there is no clinical, radiographic or electrocardiographic evidence of left ventricular enlargement or hypertrophy the murmur is unlikely to be of sufficient haemodynamic significance to warrant further investigation or restriction of activities, but an annual review would be advisable.

Coarctation of the aorta

The systolic murmur due to turbulence at the site of obstruction is usually loudest at the back over the spine but often audible anteriorly.

There may also be a systolic murmur from the frequently associated congenitally malformed aortic valve and sometimes a murmur over dilated collateral vessels.

PULMONARY SYSTOLIC MURMURS

A pulmonary systolic murmur may be due to high flow across a normal valve, to valvar stenosis, to subvalvar obstruction to RV outflow or merely to dilatation of the main pulmonary artery.

A pulmonary systolic murmur is probably the most frequent of all so-called functional or innocent murmurs.

Pulmonary stenosis

As with aortic stenosis, the characteristic murmur of pulmonary valvar stenosis is usually loudest in midsystole, corresponding with the period of maximal ejection but there is no close relationship between the intensity of the murmur and the degree of obstruction. There may be similar difficulties in precise timing. The position of the murmur in systole depends on the degree of stenosis and whether or not there is an associated ventricular septal defect providing a double outlet for the right ventricle. In general, the greater the degree of stenosis, the later the peak and the longer the duration of the murmur. There is usually a systolic thrill.

In severe pulmonary valvar stenosis the second heart sound may be widely split, but the pulmonary component is usually faint or absent, depending on the degree of obstruction, so that the sound may appear single on auscultation.

Pulmonary valvar stenosis is usually due to congenital fusion of the cusps.

Subvalvar obstruction

Subvalvar obstruction to right ventricular outflow occurs especially in one form of the congenital malformation known as Fallot's tetralogy, in which case the murmur may be loudest in the third rather than the second left intercostal space. Obstruction however may also occur from muscular hypertrophy alone or in association with valvar stenosis or a ventricular septal defect.

Increased pulmonary blood flow

A systolic murmur from increased pulmonary blood flow across a normal valve may be associated with any hyperkinetic state, such as exercise, emotion, pregnancy, anaemia or thyrotoxicosis. It is often heard in healthy young persons.

In congenital defects increased blood flow may be due to a left to right shunt from an atrial or ventricular septal defect.

A pulmonary systolic murmur is the most frequent murmur to be heard in the absence of valvar disease and the most usual cause of what used to be called a **haemic murmur** (p. 81).

In atrial septal defect the intensity of the murmur depends not only on blood flow but on dilatation of the pulmonary artery, its proximity to the chest wall and on the degree of any associated pulmonary stenosis or pulmonary hypertension. An atrial septal defect may be suspected as the cause of the murmur if the second heart sound is clearly split during expiration and 'fixed' during inspiration (p. 46).

There may also be a diastolic murmur from increased flow across the tricuspid valve (p. 97).

When due to increased flow across a normal valve the murmur tends to be more high pitched and blowing than in pulmonary stenosis. Like other right sided events it is often increased in intensity by inspiration.

Dilatation of pulmonary artery

Dilatation of the pulmonary artery with relative stenosis may occur as an isolated anomaly unassociated with heart disease and in such cases there is often a systolic murmur.

CAUSES OF MITRAL REGURGITATION

Causes

    Disease of valve cusps

    Dilatation of the annulus or left ventricular chamber

    Dysfunction or rupture of papillary muscle

    Chordal rupture

Aetiology

    Rheumatic fever

    Left ventricular failure

    Myocardial ischaemia or infarction

    Infective endocarditis

    Myocardiopathy

    Congenital malformation

    Trauma

APICAL SYSTOLIC MURMURS

An apical systolic murmur is most often due to mitral regurgitation, of which there are a number of different causes, but may be transmitted and derive from aortic valvar stenosis, subaortic obstruction to left ventricular outflow, tricuspid regurgitation, or a ventricular septal defect.

MITRAL REGURGITATION

The characteristic murmur of mitral regurgitation is pansystolic, loudest at the apex and often well heard towards the left axilla and lung base. The murmur is usually blowing or harsh in character and may be accompanied by a systolic thrill.

As with other forms of valvar disease, intensity of the murmur is an unreliable guide to the severity of the defect but severe regurgitation is likely to be present if there is also a third heart sound (p. 55) which is often followed by a short, early decrescendo diastolic flow murmur (p. 97).

Less frequently the murmur occurs in late, mid or even early systole.

The causes and aetiology of mitral regurgitation are listed in the table.

Rheumatic mitral disease

This is probably still the most frequent cause even in the Western world and usually the diagnosis is obvious. In the absence of other evidence of heart disease, the finding on routine examination of an apical systolic murmur always raises the possibility of rheumatic mitral disease and this is a frequent source of uncertainty in diagnosis. If there is a past history of rheumatic fever or radiographic evidence of enlargement of the left auricle as well as the atrium, this diagnosis must be made.

However, even if there is no other abnormality, it still cannot be denied that minimal rheumatic heart disease is present and, if possible, examination should be repeated at intervals until it is certain that the situation is stationary.

Usually it is more important to avoid the error of diagnosing organic heart disease when none is present than to ignore a minor organic murmur, and this slight risk may reasonably be taken. In the occasional instance, infective endocarditis may subsequently develop in mild rheumatic mitral disease, but on balance there can be no question that this risk also should be accepted. From the practical point of view minor rheumatic mitral regurgitation in the absence of cardiac enlargement is of little haemodynamic significance and the patient should be reassured that the heart is healthy.

Regurgitant jet in mitral stenosis

In patients with mitral stenosis, especially with a sclerotic or calcified valve, it may not be possible for the cusps to come into perfect apposition in ventricular systole with a resultant regurgitant jet. This is often of no haemodynamic importance in comparison with the degree of obstruction, and is not a contraindication to valvotomy. Such a murmur may be loud and is often high pitched or musical but usually not well conducted towards the left axilla. In such cases other physical signs denote dominant stenosis.

In other cases the relative degrees of mitral stenosis and regurgitation may be balanced or nearly so and the practical problem often arises as to whether closed valvotomy or valve replacement is indicated. The decision as to which defect is dominant can often be decided by taking in account the findings on palpation and auscultation together with radiography and electrocardiography, but sometimes cardiac catheterisation with left ventricular angiography is necessary.

Apart from the haemodynamic aspects the significance of mitral regurgitation is often largely dependent upon its aetiology.

Functional mitral regurgitation

Functional mitral regurgitation, in the correct sense of the term, that is with normal valve cusps, may result from dilatation of the valve ring or from dilatation of the left ventricular chamber with 'pulling' on the chordae and papillary muscles.

Papillary muscle dysfunction or rupture

Dysfunction of the papillary muscles commonly results from

coronary heart disease. This may occur acutely or be responsible for the finding of a mitral systolic murmur in the elderly.

Rupture of a papillary muscle may occur from acute myocardial infarction and require urgent surgical treatment. Differential diagnosis is from rupture of the interventricular septum and the distinction is important in relation to the timing of surgical treatment if this is indicated by the severity of symptoms.

Ruptured chordae tendineae

Rupture of chordae tendineae may occur spontaneously for no obvious reason or in patients with rheumatic heart disease and the regurgitant jet may be in an unusual direction. With posterior rupture it may strike the left atrial wall opposite the root of the aorta giving rise to a systolic murmur and thrill in the right upper chest. This sometimes causes difficulty in differential diagnosis from an aortic murmur and the distinction is important because surgical treatment may be indicated. With anterior rupture the jet may be in the direction of the left sternal border and the murmur simulates a ventricular septal defect.

Infective endocarditis

Infective endocarditis rarely occurs in the absence of a murmur and most frequently with mild mitral or aortic regurgitation. The condition is notably rare in severe mitral stenosis.

A change in the quality of a previously present mitral systolic murmur may provide a helpful clue when there is uncertainty as to the diagnosis of infective endocarditis. After treatment the healing process with sclerosis may result in increased severity of the valvar defect.

Congenital mitral regurgitation

Congenital mitral regurgitation is usually due to a cleft in the aortic cusp of the valve associated with maldevelopment of the endocardial cushions and a persistent ostium primum in the interatrial septum.

In a patient with signs of an atrial septal defect, a mitral systolic murmur strongly suggests that the defect is of the ostium primum variety and is therefore important in relation to surgical treatment.

Myocardiopathy

Mitral regurgitation may result from a variety of causes in myocardiopathy including distortion, papillary muscle dysfunction and cardiac failure.

Trauma

The most frequent cause of traumatic mitral regurgitation is mitral valvotomy. Rarely, rupture of a cusp or chordae results from external trauma.

TRANSMITTED MURMURS

It has already been emphasised that the murmur of aortic stenosis may be loudest at the apex and thus cause confusion in diagnosis. Despite the classical differences in timing and in quality, when aortic stenosis and mitral regurgitation are both present, differentiation by auscultation may be impossible.

Sometimes in patients with enlargement of the heart a systolic murmur from tricuspid regurgitation is loudest at the apex and may be mistaken for that of mitral regurgitation. In such cases it may be noted that the loudness of the murmur increases during and shortly after a slow, deep inspiration in contrast to the murmur of mitral regurgitation which usually decreases in intensity.

In ventricular septal defect, whether due to congenital malformation or myocardial infarction, the murmur is usually loudest at the left sternal border at about the level of the fourth rib but, if loud, may be well heard at the apex.

In small children differentiation between murmurs due to a ventricular septal defect, aortic stenosis, and mitral regurgitation may be difficult.

LEFT PARASTERNAL SYSTOLIC MURMURS

A systolic murmur which is loudest at the left sternal border is most likely to be due to one of the causes listed below.

Increased pulmonary blood flow
Obstruction to right ventricular outflow
Ventricular septal defect
Tricuspid regurgitation
Obstruction to left ventricular outflow
Idiopathic.

The clinical features of these various conditions are described under the appropriate headings.

If there is other evidence of heart disease in the form of cardiac enlargement or hypertrophy it will be important to establish the cause and, since accuracy in diagnosis is an essential prerequisite for the consideration of surgical treatment, cardiac catheterisation will often be necessary. However, the most likely cause will usually be indicated by clinical examination.

Upper sternal border

The commonest causes are increased pulmonary blood flow or obstruction to right ventricular outflow.

Sometimes only a systolic murmur is present in a patient with patency of the ductus arteriosus, either in infancy when the pulmonary vascular resistance is still relatively high, or in later life if secondary pulmonary hypertension develops.

Midsternal border

The commonest cause of a systolic murmur which is loudest in the third or fourth intercostal space is a ventricular septal defect and in such cases is often, but not invariably, accompanied by a thrill. The murmur may be pansystolic because, throughout systole, pressure in the left ventricle is greater than that in the right ventricle but can be relatively short if the pulmonary vascular resistance is raised.

A murmur which is loudest in this region may of course be transmitted from elsewhere.

Lower sternal border

A systolic murmur which is loudest in the lower sternal border may be due to tricuspid regurgitation. This may result from organic deformity of the cusps due to rheumatic endocarditis or to dilatation of the valve ring with cardiac failure due to pulmonary hypertension, especially in mitral stenosis. This murmur often increases in intensity during and shortly after deep inspiration (p. 94).

A loud systolic murmur from a neighbouring region may also be audible here.

Isolated 'vibratory' parasternal murmur

A left lower parasternal systolic murmur without any other abnormality to suggest heart disease is a frequent finding in youth and often has a characteristic vibratory quality. In such cases the best term to use is 'idiopathic'.

COMMENT ON TERMINOLOGY

The term 'functional' is often used to signify the presence of a murmur in the absence of any evidence of structural abnormality. However, functional is also frequently used when a murmur from mitral or tricuspid regurgitation is secondary to dilatation of the valve ring rather than to organic disease of the cusps. It is therefore better avoided as an alternative to 'innocent'.

The term 'innocent' is likewise open to objection because it is not always possible to be certain from a single examination that an apparently innocent systolic murmur is not due to mild organic disease, or, of course, that such disease may not in time be progressive. For example a faint aortic systolic murmur may be based on a congenital bicuspid valve which in later life will become calcified and narrow.

Likewise, a faint apical systolic murmur may be due to rheumatic valvitis with slight regurgitation to be followed in due course by mitral stenosis or by infective endocarditis.

Nevertheless, there are occasions when the term 'innocent' is justified, as, for example, when applied to the pulmonary systolic murmur so often present in healthy children or during pregnancy. A similar murmur may be due to increased blood flow from anaemia or thyrotoxicosis.

'*Isolated*' may be used when there is no other evidence of heart disease and '*idiopathic*' when the cause is obscure.

The chief danger is usually that of engendering anxiety when a murmur is found as an isolated anomaly in the absence of other evidence of heart disease. It is very important to avoid this and also the imposition of unwarranted restrictions. Infants and children must be kept under observation and examined at intervals because, at this age, it is often impossible to be certain as to the nature of a systolic murmur.

In young adults it is best to arrange for re-examination after, say, 12 months, but at the same time to give reassurance that no restrictions in activity are indicated and that a normal life can be led in every way.

In older patients an isolated systolic murmur can more readily be ignored, but again it should be remembered that in youth an aortic systolic murmur may signify valvar stenosis which does not become of haemodynamic significance until quite late in life, for example after the age of 50. In the elderly, common causes for unimportant systolic murmurs are sclerosis of the aortic valve or calcification of the mitral ring. Papillary muscle dysfunction is another cause of mild mitral regurgitation and its significance is dependent upon that of associated coronary heart disease.

Haemic murmur

The term 'haemic murmur' is best avoided in that it only signifies a murmur associated with a hyperkinetic circulation. In the majority of such cases the murmur is that of increased pulmonary blood flow but, on occasion, with severe anaemia, there may be dilatation of the valve ring with functional mitral regurgitation.

In all cases it is best to state, when possible, the site of origin of the murmur or, when this cannot be ascertained, to use the term 'idiopathic'.

There is no harm in using the term 'isolated' when there is no other abnormality to be found, but in such cases one of the other terms referred to above is usually preferable.

Ejection murmur

The term 'ejection murmur' has served a useful purpose in drawing attention to the value of precise timing of systolic murmurs and the conclusions of practical significance which can be drawn. On the other hand, it has now outlived its usefulness and paradoxically led to confusion, not only from misuse, for which blame can only be attached to the observer, but because the term is not always accurate as regards its conventional implications.

It was introduced to signify a murmur produced at the aortic or pulmonary valve which began shortly after the first heart sound, reached its maximum in midsystole and ceased before the second sound. Its phonocardiographic configuration is described as being that of a diamond.

By contrast other systolic murmurs including those from mitral or tricuspid regurgitation or from a ventricular septal defect were said to be pansystolic or holosystolic, that is to say, beginning with the first heart sound and lasting throughout systole up to and occasionally beyond one component of the second sound.

Undoubtedly murmurs do frequently have the characteristics described which are useful in diagnosis, but there are numerous exceptions.

Objections to 'ejection'. Although blood is 'ejected' from the ventricular cavity into the aorta or pulmonary artery, likewise it is ejected through an incompetent mitral or tricuspid valve or from one ventricle to another through a septal defect. It is not therefore a very meaningful term.

Precise timing is not always easy to judge by auscultation because frequently one or other or both heart sounds cannot be heard.

The configuration of an aortic or pulmonary systolic murmur varies. It may start early in systole or commence relatively late and is not always loudest in midsystole. In some degree apparent duration is influenced by intensity. Even on the phonocardiogram the 'diamond' is often pretty rough.

The qualities of the murmur depend on whether it is due to increased blood flow or to obstruction. If due to obstruction it depends on the area of the valve and the gradient across it which in turn depends on a number of factors including the force of ventricular contraction, the stroke volume, the duration of systole and the pressure in the aorta or pulmonary artery.

A pulmonary systolic murmur from increased flow will be influenced by pulmonary hypertension and one from stenosis, not only by its degree but by whether or not there is a ventricular septal defect.

A systolic murmur from mitral regurgitation is often long, but sometimes relatively short, and sometimes loudest in midsystole or sometimes late.

The murmur of a ventricular septal defect will be relatively short if there is pulmonary hypertension.

An aortic systolic murmur may be loudest at the left sternal border or even at the apex of the heart and a mitral systolic murmur, as when due to ruptured chordae, may be loudest in the conventional aortic area.

The qualities of an aortic systolic murmur do not always seem the same at the upper sternal right border, the mid-left sternal border, or at the apex, although timing is similar.

In a patient with both aortic stenosis and mitral regurgitation it is not always possible to distinguish the two components of an apical systolic murmur by auscultation.

Unfortunately any murmur found in the aortic or pulmonary area tends to be described as an ejection murmur and most apical systolic murmurs are described as pansystolic.

Additional points which have led to confusion are that there are other systolic murmurs with the qualities usually attributed to an 'ejection' murmur which are not derived at the aortic or pulmonary valve; for example the murmur of subvalvar obstruction, and many so-called 'innocent' parasternal murmurs which are not associated with any evidence of heart disease and for which the explanation is obscure.

At the present time errors are made through using a classification which is convenient and often accurate but sometimes misleading through making unwarranted assumptions and paying relatively little attention to precise timing and characteristics. It is for all these reasons that it would be better abandoned.

The alternative is to determine and record the precise characteristics in each patient and make appropriate deductions from a summation of all available evidence including palpation.

APPROACH TO AN ISOLATED SYSTOLIC MURMUR

An isolated systolic murmur may be due to increased blood flow across a normal valve, to valvar disease, to an intra- or extra-cardiac shunt or to vascular narrowing. Attention should be paid to its site of maximal intensity, radiation, loudness, timing, duration and quality, the effect of changes of posture and respiration, the presence or absence of a thrill, and any abnormality of the heart sounds. An isolated systolic murmur, that is to say with normal heart sounds and in the absence of a thrill, diastolic murmur, cardiac enlargement, hypertrophy or failure, and with a normal X-ray and E.C.G., can usually be ignored and the patient reassured. Sometimes, as indicated above, a review at intervals is wise. An occasional error may be made by ignoring such a murmur but the risk of this is much less than that of engendering anxiety or imposing unwarranted restrictions.

EXTRACARDIAC MURMURS

Extracardiac murmurs, other than those due to pericarditis, often cause confusion to the inexperienced observer. They may be pericardial or pleuropericardial in origin, even in the absence of inflammation, but from the clinical aspect it is not always possible to be certain as to precise methods of production. They are usually different in quality from murmurs due to heart disease and are often more easy to recognise than describe. Their importance lies in lack of serious significance.

A cardiorespiratory murmur is systolic in time and varies regularly with inspiration. This murmur does not have the characteristics of organic heart disease and is probably due to compression of the expanded lung by the heart during inspiration.

In all such conditions the patient appears well and there is no evidence for any structural abnormality of the heart.

Pericardial friction

A pericardial rub is caused by friction between the visceral and parietal layers and has a characteristic, superficial, scratching quality which, in the appropriate setting, can usually be recognised. It is notoriously variable in situation and in intensity from time to time and even from hour to hour, and hence must be assiduously sought in a patient complaining of acute pain in the chest for which the cause is not obvious.

Precise timing of the components is also variable and the 'rub' may be triphasic, biphasic or monophasic, and sometimes is better heard during inspiration or expiration. Coarse pericardial friction may be palpable.

Pericardial friction may be mistaken for the 'to-and-fro' systolic and diastolic murmurs of aortic valvar disease and may be simulated by other extracardiac sounds.

It may be heard in a wide variety of clinical conditions including rheumatic fever, acute myocardial infarction, the post-myocardial infarction syndrome, tuberculosis, rheumatoid arthritis, gout, lupus erythematosus, uraemia, neoplastic invasion, pyogenic infection and after pericardiotomy. Less frequent causes include myxoedema, X-ray therapy, serum sickness, drug hypersensitivity, vaccination, fungal infection, parasitic infection, trauma to the chest wall and penetrating wounds.

CLASSIFICATION OF DIASTOLIC MURMURS

Early
> Aortic regurgitation
> Pulmonary regurgitation

Mid
1. Obstruction
   Mitral stenosis
   Tricuspid stenosis
2. Increased flow
   Mitral
   > Mitral regurgitation
   > Patent ductus arteriosus
   > Ventricular septal defect

   Tricuspid
   > Tricuspid regurgitation
   > Atrial septal defect

Late (presystolic)
> Mitral stenosis
> Tricuspid stenosis

DIASTOLIC MURMURS

Diastolic murmurs fall between the second and first heart sounds and always signify the presence of organic heart disease.

They may be due to:

1. Deformity of the valve cusps
2. Dilatation of the valve ring
3. Increased blood flow.

On the basis of timing they can be classified into three groups:

1. *Early*—beginning with the second sound and due to regurgitant flow through the aortic or pulmonary valve.

2. *Mid*—beginning a short interval after semilunar valve closure (and therefore not precisely in mid-diastole) and due to forward flow through the mitral or tricuspid valve.

3. *Late*—beginning in presystole or from apparent accentuation of a murmur starting earlier in diastole, and dependent on atrial contraction.

AORTIC REGURGITATION

Aetiology

Aortic regurgitation may arise from deformity or disease of the valve cusps or from dilatation of the valve ring and may be due to congenital or acquired defects.

Congenital: Bicuspid aortic valve
Imperfect closure of valve
Infective endocarditis
Coarctation of the aorta
Aortic stenosis with rigid cusps
Fenestration of the cusps
Marfan's disease
High ventricular septal defect
Aneurysm of sinus of Valsalva

Acquired: Rheumatic
Syphilitic
Infective endocarditis
Dissecting aneurysm
Rheumatoid arthritis
Spondylitis
Disseminated lupus erythematosus
Traumatic
Hypertension
Atherosclerosis
Leaking prosthetic valve

EARLY DIASTOLIC MURMURS

AORTIC REGURGITATION

The diastolic murmur of aortic regurgitation is usually loudest in the third and fourth intercostal spaces, close to the left sternal border. If loud it may also be heard at the apex, in which case it can usually be appreciated that there is no gap between the second sound and the beginning of the murmur. This is in contrast to the diastolic murmur of mitral stenosis when there is a distinct gap and often a preceding opening snap, as discussed on p. 93.

The murmur of aortic regurgitation is best heard with a diaphragm chest piece and with the patient sitting up or standing and with the breath held in expiration. It is well to remember these points if quiet murmurs are not to be overlooked. The murmur is usually high-pitched and blowing in quality.

If harsh or musical, and especially if heard best to the right rather than to the left of the sternum, causes other than rheumatic fever should be considered. These include rupture of an aortic cusp, infective endocarditis, syphilis, leaking aneurysm of a sinus of Valsalva and rupture of a dissecting aneurysm with dilatation of the valve ring. Occasionally a similar murmur may be heard when there is gross dilatation of the ascending aorta immediately above the valve. Differentiation can usually be made by consideration of associated circumstances.

Although in general a loud murmur will be associated with severe regurgitation, there is no close correlation between these two features and many striking discrepancies. The severity of valvar regurgitation cannot in fact be assessed by auscultation but only by examination of the peripheral circulation and by seeking evidence of left ventricular enlargement or hypertrophy. However, the signs of aortic regurgitation are often modified by associated valvar stenosis, by left ventricular failure or by other valvar defects.

With free regurgitation there will be a full, bounding 'water hammer' pulse and muscle 'knock' and a low diastolic blood pressure with a high systolic pressure and therefore high pulse pressure. Exaggerated arterial pulsations may be obvious in the carotid and other arteries and capillary pulsation in the nail beds or in the retinal vessels. A 'pistol' shot may be heard over a medium-sized vessel, such as the brachial or femoral artery, if the vessel is lightly compressed with the bell of the stethoscope. Nevertheless, especially from the surgical point of view, severe regurgitation in association with stenosis, may be present without these signs.

The actual *causes of regurgitation* include contraction of the cusps, dilatation of the valve ring, erosion or rupture of a cusp, separation of the commissures and congenital malformation.

Many of these conditions are now amenable to surgical treatment and therefore precision in diagnosis is important.

Aetiology

It is helpful to keep in mind the various conditions which may give rise to aortic regurgitation (p. 88).

The younger the patient the more likely is the defect to be due to congenital malformation.

Rheumatic fever is the most frequent cause, in which case there is often associated mitral disease.

In aortic stenosis the valve is often rigid and the cusps do not come into perfect apposition during diastole so that some degree of regurgitation is frequent, even with severe stenosis.

Infective endocarditis usually affects an already abnormal valve from congenital malformation or rheumatic fever.

Syphilis, although now uncommon, should be remembered in isolated aortic regurgitation, especially in middle-aged and younger men.

A congenital bicuspid valve is a common anomaly but more often gives rise to stenosis than regurgitation.

A high ventricular septal defect, that is to say in the membranous septum, is situated just below the aortic valve and in consequence a cusp may be unsupported.

Features of the Marfan syndrome should be sought in cases of obscure aetiology.

Downward dissection of an aortic aneurysm may be responsible for an early diastolic murmur in a patient with the sudden onset of pain in the chest.

Likewise, the sudden onset of dyspnoea may be due to rupture of an aneurysm of a sinus of Valsalva. If this is into a right sided cardiac chamber a continuous murmur is usual but if into the left ventricle, there may only be a diastolic murmur.

Disorders of connective tissue sometimes also involve the root of the aorta or valve cusps.

Severe systemic hypertension and atherosclerosis of the aorta, which often occur together, are occasional causes for mild aortic regurgitation.

Nowadays a leaking prosthetic valve has become a relatively common cause and may require further operation, often on account of haemolysis.

PULMONARY REGURGITATION

An early diastolic murmur from pulmonary regurgitation was first described by Graham-Steell in a patient with severe pulmonary hypertension from mitral stenosis. This murmur is similar in quality to that of aortic regurgitation and likewise audible down the left sternal border. It is impossible to distinguish the two by auscultation and the probability as to which valve is at fault must be decided by seeking signs of aortic regurgitation in the peripheral circulation on the one hand and those of pulmonary hypertension on the other.

Pulmonary hypertension will be indicated by a loud pulmonary component of the second heart sound, by clinical or electrocardiographic evidence of right ventricular hypertrophy and by radiographic enlargement of the main pulmonary artery and its first two branches. However, it is not possible to diagnose a Graham-Steell murmur with certainty before operation because, in patients with mitral stenosis, associated mild aortic regurgitation, that is without peripheral signs, is frequent. If, following valvotomy, the early diastolic murmur disappears then, in retrospect, the diagnosis can be made with confidence.

Pulmonary regurgitation may also occur with gross dilatation of the pulmonary artery from any cause including isolated, idiopathic dilatation.

PULMONARY REGURGITATION

Aetiology

Congenital causes: Bicuspid valve
Other malformation of cusps
Dilatation of pulmonary artery
Pulmonary stenosis
Pulmonary hypertension

Acquired causes: Pulmonary hypertension
Mitral disease
Pulmonary heart disease
Massive pulmonary embolism

Surgical treatment for valvar stenosis

Miscellaneous rarities
Rheumatic fever, syphilis, infective endo-carditis, carcinoid syndrome and external trauma

MID-DIASTOLIC MURMURS

A mid-diastolic murmur may be heard in mitral or tricuspid stenosis or with increased flow across the valve without stenosis.

Actually 'mid' is not strictly accurate with regard to valvar stenosis because the murmur starts a short interval after the second sound immediately following the opening snap of the mitral or tricuspid valve. However, merely to call it a mitral diastolic murmur does not distinguish it from a presystolic murmur and the term is therefore convenient.

The causes are listed in the table on page 86.

Mitral stenosis

The cardinal sign of mitral stenosis is a long, rumbling, diastolic murmur, loudest at, or localised to, the apex. If, as is so often the case, atrial fibrillation is present, there will be no presystolic accentuation.

This murmur is best heard or may only be heard if the patient is lying down and turned towards the left side, or if blood flow is increased by exercise. These manoeuvres should therefore be part of the routine examination of any patient suspected of having mitral disease.

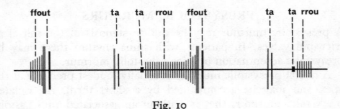

Fig. 10

The *classical* signs of mitral stenosis are a loud, slapping, first heart sound preceded by a crescendo presystolic murmur and an opening snap followed by a rumbling, mid-diastolic murmur. This cadence gives rise to the onomatopoeic 'ffout ta ta rrou' first described by Duroziez (Fig. 10).

The first or presystolic element of this sequence occurs late in ventricular diastole, synchronous with the forceful passage of blood into the ventricle produced by atrial systole. This presystolic accentuation is only heard in patients with sinus rhythm and disappears with the onset of fibrillation. It is incorrect to say that the *presystolic murmur* disappears because the diastolic murmur continues up to the first sound and it is only the crescendo accentuation which is absent in atrial fibrillation.

It used to be thought that a mitral diastolic murmur at the apex was diagnostic of obstruction but, with the increased precision in auscultation which came with phonocardiography, and, in particular, the stimulus to careful auscultation brought by the advent of cardiac surgery, it has been recognised that a murmur, similar in time but different in origin, may occur in patients with increased blood flow across the valve. Such conditions include mitral regurgitation, ventricular septal defect and patent ductus arteriosus, and are discussed below.

Tricuspid stenosis

The diastolic murmur of tricuspid stenosis is best heard to the left of the lower sternal border or nearer the apex and becomes loudest during, and immediately after, deep inspiration owing to increased right atrial filling from the great veins. It is not usually rumbling in quality as is the diastolic murmur of mitral stenosis.

PRESYSTOLIC MURMURS

A presystolic murmur may be due to stenosis of the mitral or tricuspid valves. In patients with sinus rhythm there may be presystolic accentuation of a long diastolic murmur.

A mitral presystolic murmur is usually loudest precisely at the apex and may be accompanied by a short thrill. An isolated presystolic murmur, that is without an associated mid-diastolic murmur, is only found in the early or mild stages of mitral stenosis.

A presystolic murmur, similar in quality to mitral stenosis, may be heard with tricuspid stenosis. This possibility should always be considered in patients with signs of mitral disease, especially if the presystolic murmur is very clear, well heard towards the sternum and is louder in deep inspiration, which increases blood flow across the tricuspid valve. In such cases there is likely to be a prominent 'a' wave in the jugular venous pulse and a peaked 'P' wave in the electrocardiogram.

Austin Flint murmur

Austin Flint originally described a presystolic murmur in a patient with aortic regurgitation but without mitral disease. However, it has become customary in such cases to use this eponym for any apical diastolic murmur simulating that of mitral stenosis but without other evidence for it.

In patients with aortic regurgitation of non-rheumatic aetiology, such as syphilis, this murmur may be diagnosed with reasonable confidence, but in those with rheumatic heart disease it is guess work and in any case the distinction is more of academic than practical importance. Nevertheless, the genesis of such a murmur is of interest and a number of theories have been proposed, any of which may be operative in different cases. These include:

Displacement of the anterior leaflet of the mitral valve towards the atrium by the regurgitant stream from the aortic valve producing functional mitral stenosis. This murmur is due to forward flow.

Reversal of the LV-LA gradient producing diastolic mitral regurgitation. This murmur is due to backward flow and has been shown in some cases by cardiac catheterisation and cine-angiocardiography.

Vibrations of the aortic leaflet of the mitral valve between the two streams of blood.

Mitral regurgitation may also result from dilatation of the left ventricle or the AV ring.

APICAL DIASTOLIC MURMURS

Aetiology

Mitral stenosis

Increased mitral flow
   Mitral regurgitation
   Ventricular septal defect
   Patent ductus arteriosus

Mitral valvitis (Carey Coombs murmur)

Austin Flint murmur

Transmission of other murmurs
   Aortic regurgitation
   Pulmonary regurgitation
   Tricuspid stenosis
   Increased tricuspid flow

Coarctation of the aorta

APICAL DIASTOLIC MURMURS

An apical diastolic murmur is most frequently due to mitral stenosis but may also occur in a number of other conditions including increased blood flow across the mitral valve and transmission from other areas.

In the acute stage of mitral valvitis there may be a transient, short, diastolic murmur, as first described by Carey Coombs. It is probably due to oedema of the cusps.

In severe mitral regurgitation, owing to increased blood flow across the valve, there is often a decrescendo murmur in mid-diastole which begins abruptly and usually after a third heart sound.

In ventricular septal defect and patency of the ductus arteriosus there may be a similar diastolic murmur from increased flow together with characteristic signs of the primary condition.

The murmurs of aortic and pulmonary regurgitation begin early after the second sound and are usually loudest at the left sternal border but may be well heard at the apex.

In isolated aortic regurgitation there may be a mitral diastolic murmur, as first described by Austin Flint.

In tricuspid stenosis and with increased tricuspid flow, as from a large atrial septal defect with considerable cardiac enlargement, the diastolic murmur may be loudest at the apex.

In coarctation of the aorta an apical diastolic murmur is occasionally present and probably attributable to relative mitral stenosis from dilatation of the left ventricle.

CONTINUOUS MURMURS

Causes

1. Patent ductus arteriosus
2. Aortic-pulmonary window
3. Ruptured sinus of Valsalva
4. Coronary arteriovenous fistula
5. Bronchopulmonary arterial anastomoses
6. Pulmonary arterial branch stenosis
7. Pulmonary arteriovenous fistula
8. Common truncus arteriosus
9. Total anomalous pulmonary venous drainage
10. Coarctation of the aorta
11. Aortic stenosis plus aortic regurgitation
12. Ventricular septal defect plus aortic regurgitation
13. Venous hum
14. Mammary souffle
15. Traumatic AV fistula
16. Palliative surgical treatment with creation of a shunt
17. Miscellaneous rarities

CONTINUOUS MURMURS

A continuous murmur is one which begins in systole and continues through the second sound into diastole. It is usually due to blood flowing from a high to a low pressure chamber or vessel and hence to some form of arteriovenous communication. However, it may also result from disturbances of flow in a narrowed vessel.

The precise configuration of a continuous murmur, as judged by ear or phonocardiography, is variable and depends on local circumstances.

Aetiology

The chief causes of a continuous murmur are listed in the table.

Patency of the ductus arteriosus is by far the most frequent cause and was first described by Dr Gibson of Edinburgh. It has a characteristic 'machinery-like' quality with accentuation in late systole when the gradient is greatest and is loudest in the second left intercostal space.

In infancy only a systolic murmur may be present because of the relatively high pressure in the pulmonary artery. Likewise, if in later years pulmonary hypertension develops, the diastolic part of the murmur shortens and finally disappears. Later the systolic part may also be abbreviated and in some cases, when the pressures are balanced no murmur may be audible.

Surgical treatment is usually advised because of the risk of infective endocarditis or, in later years, of cardiac failure.

An aortopulmonary fistula just above the valves is a similar but much rarer condition and more liable to be associated with pulmonary hypertension. It cannot be distinguished with certainty except by cardiac catheterisation but if this were carried out as a routine very many patients would have an unnecessary procedure for the sake of picking up a very occasional case.

There are numerous other causes of a continuous murmur, and accuracy of diagnosis is important not only to avoid an inappropriate operation but because definitive treatment for the causative condition may be necessary. However, it will be appreciated from the above table that if due consideration is given to all associated clinical, radiographic and electrocardiographic features, errors should be uncommon and the indications for more specialised investigation will usually be clear.

Arteriovenous fistulae may be congenital or acquired. They are sometimes due to surgical treatment as when a palliative operation is carried out for certain forms of severe congenital heart disease with the deliberate creation of a shunt. The commonest example is for Fallot's tetralogy.

The murmur associated with a pulmonary arteriovenous fistula is usually systolic and heard over the lower lobe of the lung, but occasionally it is continuous. In these cases there will also be central cyanosis and clubbing of the fingers.

Examples of continuous murmurs due to a disturbance of flow in a narrowed segment include coarctation of the aorta, pulmonary arterial branch stenosis and, rarely, pulmonary embolism with partial occlusion of the vessel.

Continuous murmurs from disturbances of flow may also occur with bronchial arterial collateral vessels and with collaterals from coarctation of the aorta.

A high ventricular septal defect in the membranous part of the septum may result in an aortic cusp being unsupported with consequent valvar regurgitation. In such cases the murmur is almost continuous, but in the more frequent combination of aortic stenosis and regurgitation there is a distinct, if slight, gap and the murmur is more reasonably described as being 'to and fro' in quality.

A mammary souffle is not uncommon over the lactating breast.

Venous hum

A venous hum is a physiological flow murmur which may be heard at the root of the neck in many children and in some young adults. It is continuous with accentuation during diastole, increases on inspiration and is usually loudest on the right side with the subject sitting or standing. It diminishes or disappears on recumbency.

Light pressure with the stethoscope accentuates the murmur and firmer pressure abolishes it. If heard below the clavicle it may simulate a patent ductus but can be abolished by light pressure with the finger over the jugular vein, or may be modified by turning the head. The importance of a venous hum lies only in its recognition and possible misinterpretation for some other form of arteriovenous communication.

ACUTE MYOCARDIAL INFARCTION

Complications

1. Sudden death
   Ventricular fibrillation
   Ventricular asystole
   Weak ineffectual contractions
2. Pulmonary oedema
3. Shock
4. Triple rhythm
5. Bradycardia
6. Dysrhythmias
7. Defects of conduction
8. Pericarditis
9. Pulmonary embolism
10. Systemic embolism
11. Papillary muscle dysfunction or rupture
12. Rupture of ventricular septum or free wall
13. Congestive failure
14. Ventricular aneurysm

SUMMARIES OF COMMONEST DISORDERS

The following summaries describe the classical clinical features of fairly severe defects, but it will be appreciated that all grades of severity may occur and often combinations of defects.

ACUTE MYOCARDIAL INFARCTION

It would be inappropriate here to describe in detail the clinical manifestations of acute myocardial infarction and its complications, but certain bedside observations in addition to auscultation may be of critical importance, especially in the absence of facilities for monitoring. Early recognition and appropriate management may be life-saving.

The onset of myocardial infarction is usually sudden with collapse, chest pain or dyspnoea.

Cardiac pain may be simulated by various conditions including:

Acute pericarditis
Massive pulmonary embolism
Dissecting aneurysm of the aorta
Oesophageal and upper abdominal disorders
Skeletal conditions involving the lower cervical and upper
thoracic spine.

Sudden death is frequent and often the first manifestation of coronary heart disease. The commonest cause is ventricular fibrillation and, if facilities for electrical defibrillation are not immediately available, first aid measures should be instituted and continued until appropriate treatment can be given.

Asystole requires electrical pacing.

Ineffectual contractions reflect myocardial failure, for which little at present can be done.

Dyspnoea from pulmonary congestion or oedema is due to left ventricular failure. This may be indicated by crepitations, but routine radiography has shown that pulmonary oedema may be present without abnormal signs in the lungs.

The signs of *shock* are due to a low cardiac output with hypotension and compensatory vasoconstriction. They include a cold clammy skin with a rapid thready pulse and often apathy, restlessness and mental confusion.

Triple rhythm, especially from the addition of a presystolic (atrial) sound, is commonly present and may be palpable, especially if the patient is turned on to the left side. Sometimes it is the first sound to be detected and suggests myocardial infarction as the explanation for otherwise unexplained symptoms.

The most frequent *dysrhythmias* are ventricular extrasystoles, ventricular tachycardia, atrial fibrillation and atrial tachycardia, but often an E.C.G. is necessary for certain diagnosis.

Sinus bradycardia often precedes heart block or ventricular dysrhythmias, and should invariably be treated.

Pericarditis will be recognised by hearing a rub and may account for the reappearance of pain.

Papillary muscle dysfunction is indicated by the development of an apical systolic murmur. If accompanied by acute symptoms, muscle rupture is probable and may require surgical treatment.

Rupture of the ventricular septum is indicated by the development of a parasternal systolic murmur and rupture of the free wall by collapse and early death. The former can be treated surgically but not in the acute stage.

Congestive failure is used for want of a better term and indicates the familiar clinical picture of peripheral oedema, a raised jugular venous pressure and engorgement of the liver, but pulmonary oedema is also 'congestive'. In the present text it is basically due to left ventricular myocardial failure with fluid retention.

Abnormal systolic pulsation in the acute stage of myocardial infarction is frequently present from left ventricular dysfunction The later development of a similar pulsation may be due to a ventricular aneurysm which may often be diagnosed with greater certainty by palpation than by radiography or radioscopy.

Massive pulmonary embolism is characterised by the sudden onset of respiratory distress with hyperventilation, cyanosis and anxiety. Sometimes cardiac pain is also present from myocardial ischaemia due to acute coronary insufficiency. Lesser embolism may only be recognised by the appearance of pleural pain or haemoptysis.

Systemic embolism may result from thrombus formation on the ventricular endocardium.

MASSIVE PULMONARY EMBOLISM

The symptoms of massive pulmonary embolism develop suddenly and are mainly due to circulatory obstruction with a fall in cardiac output. Pulmonary infarction may or may not follow.

Often there is a suggestive clinical setting for its development such as thrombophlebtitis, the onset of an arrhythmia, a recent operation or pregnancy, unaccustomed bedrest, especially for some debilitating disease, or cardiac failure.

The characteristic features are acute respiratory distress with anxiety, hyperpnoea and a rapid pulse of small volume. Cyanosis may be intense. Sometimes there is pain from myocardial ischaemia but more often a sensation of oppression in the chest.

The jugular venous pressure is raised and the systemic arterial pressure falls. Triple rhythm is often audible from the addition of a presystolic or early diastolic sound.

The pulmonary component of the second heart sound may or may not be loud depending on the cardiac output.

Occasionally a tricuspid systolic or pulmonary diastolic murmur develops.

In severe cases there may be loss of consciousness or the clinical picture of shock, the patient becoming pale, cold and clammy with a weak thready pulse.

Usually there is considerable apprehension and a sensation of impending disaster which is often fulfilled.

Retrosternal pain with the clinical picture of shock may lead to an erroneous diagnosis of myocardial infarction. Fortunately, initial treatment is essentially the same unless facilities for pulmonary embolectomy are available.

The signs of pulmonary infarction include pleuritic pain, fever and haemoptysis, but the latter sympton is often absent. Jaundice may follow, due to the breaking down of haemoglobin, in which case urobilinogen will be present in the urine. Pleural friction may be heard and an effusion sometimes develops.

PULMONARY HYPERTENSION

Pulmonary hypertension is suggested by a loud pulmonary component of the second heart sound, palpable pulmonary valve closure, and evidence of right ventricular (RV) hypertrophy. However, there is no close relationship between the degree of pulmonary hypertension (PHT) and the loudness of the second sound.

There may be physical signs of various forms of congenital or acquired heart disease but occasionally the condition may be present without obvious cause (primary pulmonary hypertension).

Other signs include a presystolic triple rhythm from atrial contraction against resistance, a pulmonary systolic murmur and ejection click and an early diastolic murmur from pulmonary regurgitation. In advanced cases with cardiac failure there may be a third heart sound from right ventricular failure and a systolic murmur from functional tricuspid regurgitation. In addition, the pulse may be of small volume with peripheral cyanosis from a low cardiac output.

The detection of PHT is of importance in all cases in which it is present because it indicates the necessity for establishing a precise diagnosis with a view to appropriate treatment. This may require radiography, electrocardiography and sometimes more elaborate laboratory methods. Likewise, in a negative sense, the *absence* of PHT in a patient with heart disease liable to be associated with it is reassuring, and will often obviate the need for more elaborate methods of investigation.

Congenital conditions are mainly those with a left to right shunt and the principal acquired causes are mitral disease, left ventricular failure, chronic pulmonary disease and massive or recurrent pulmonary embolism.

CARDIAC COMPRESSION

Compression of the heart may result from pericardial fluid or constrictive pericarditis.

The term cardiac tamponade signifies acute compression by an increase in intrapericardial pressure due to haemorrhage or effusion.

The haemodynamic effects of compression are impairment of diastolic filling and consequently of myocardial contraction. As a result stroke volume is reduced and, above a critical level of intrapericardial pressure, the cardiac output falls.

Cardiac tamponade

The amount of fluid which must accumulate before haemo-dynamic effects are noticable depends on its rate of formation and the distensibility of the pericardial sac. A large effusion may accumulate slowly with no more than a slight rise in jugular venous pressure. On the other hand acute tamponade may result from a small effusion of rapid development. The situation is clearly an emergency one with the patient distressed, dyspnoeic, apprehensive and complaining of a feeling of oppression in the chest but not actual pain. The most favoured posture is sitting forward with elbows supported, but true orthopnoea is absent.

The principal signs are due to a fall in cardiac output and in systemic arterial pressure with a compensatory rise in systemic venous pressure and tachycardia.

The deep neck veins are engorged with exaggerated pulsation and there may be a paradoxical increase in venous pressure during inspiration, that is to say, the reverse of normal. The radial pulse is rapid and of low volume and characteristically pulsus paradoxus is present, that is to say, there is an un-mistakable fall in volume during inspiration (p. 11). Peripheral cyanosis may be present but there is no oedema.

The characteristic cardiac signs are in effect negative ones, that is to say, there may be no evidence of heart disease in the form of cardiac enlargement or hypertrophy and no abnormal sounds or murmurs. There may be muffling or damping of the heart sounds.

Accurate diagnosis is important because paracentesis may be life saving. Removal of only a few mm of fluid may be followed by dramatic relief.

Aetiological factors to be considered include tuberculosis, viral infection, neoplasm and haemorrhage from trauma or dissecting aneurysm. Other causes of pericarditis are unlikely to result in acute compression.

BEDSIDE APPROACH TO TACHYCARDIA OR DYSRHYTHMIAS

Although in practice a brief history will first be taken, when the problem is one of acute dysrhythmia or defect of conduction this aspect will necessarily be limited. However, enquiry should be made as to whether the patient is being treated with digitalis or oral diuretics and as regards a previous history of similar attacks.

The radial pulse should be felt for rate and rhythm and the jugular venous pulse inspected for atrial waves which may be irregular or more rapid than ventricular waves and for cannon waves which indicate AV dissociation or AV junctional (nodal) rhythm. Cannon waves with bradycardia suggest complete heart block and with tachycardia a ventricular dysrhythmia.

Auscultation will confirm rate and rhythm and reveal any pulse deficit, and there may be signs of valvar disease. Variation in the intensity of the first heart sound, if not due to atrial fibrillation, suggests AV dissociation. If only a single sound can be heard ventricular tachycardia is a probable cause of a rapid rate. Clear splitting of the heart sounds also suggest ventricular tachycardia.

Palpation of the chest wall may reveal evidence of heart disease in the form of cardiac enlargement of hypertrophy or a thrill.

Carotid sinus massage may terminate an attack of atrial tachycardia, will have no effect on ventricular tachycardia and may temporarily slow the ventricular rate in atrial flutter.

Extrasystoles

Extrasystoles are characterised by a regular rhythm which is interrupted by premature beats followed by relatively long (compensatory) pauses. However, if multiple extrasystole are present the condition stimulate atrial fibrillation. In most cases they disappear or become less frequent with exercise. The heart sounds vary in intensity with the duration of the preceding diastole.

Occasional extrasystoles are very common in healthy individuals but may be the cause of palpitation.

They may also be associated with any form of heart disease and usually their significance is entirely that of the severity of the underlying condition. However, in acute myocardial infarction, they may precede a more serious dysrhythmia even in relatively mild cases as judged by the severity of myocardial damage, that is to say, they are due to an electrical disturbance involving the cell membrane.

Atrial fibrillation

Atrial fibrillation should be suspected when the heart beat and radial pulse are totally irregular in time and force.

The condition must be distinguished from multiple extra-systoles and from atrial flutter or tachycardia with varying block.

It may be difficult to be certain of the diagnosis, especially if the ventricular rate is relatively slow, or impossible if there is associated heart block.

Owing to the irregular duration of cardiac cycles the intensity of heart sounds and the duration of murmurs vary from beat to beat.

The most frequent causes of fibrillation should be kept in mind and confirmatory signs sought. These include rheumatic heart disease, coronary heart disease, thyrotoxicosis, myocarditis and myocardiopathy, constrictive pericarditis and neoplastic invasion. In acute conditions it may result from myocardial infarction, massive pulmonary embolism, thoracotomy, external trauma, electrocution and other rarities. Transient attacks may be precipitated by emotional stimuli or other causes for catecholamine secretion.

It may also occur without obvious cause as an isolated anomaly and persistent or recur over many years. However, in some cases signs of coronary heart disease, such as thyrotoxicosis or some other relevant condition, appear in time.

Atrial flutter

Atrial flutter should be suspected if the heart rate is about 160/minute and flutter waves can be seen in the jugular venous pulse, or if there is temporary ventricular slowing with carotid sinus pressure.

The ventricular rate may be regular or, if there is varying AV block, irregular.

The aetiology of flutter is much the same as for atrial fibrillation but the condition is less frequent.

Atrial tachycardia

Regular atrial tachycardia is usually at a rate of about 160/minute and most frequently occurs in the absence of any other detectable abnormality but may be a complication of heart disease. It is often due to digitalis intoxication, especially with hypokalaemia due to oral diuretics. Since this condition may be fatal if unrecognised accurate diagnosis by electrocardiography is important and urgent.

Atrial tachycardia can often be terminated by carotid sinus massage and especially, in resistant cases, after the administration of digitalis.

Ventricular tachycardia

Ventricular tachycardia is due to the rapid discharge of an ectopic focus in one or other ventricle. As a result ventricular contractions are asynchronous and splitting of the heart sounds occurs.

Carotid sinus massage has no effect on this dysrhythmia.

MITRAL STENOSIS

The classical signs are a loud first sound, opening snap and rumbling diastolic murmur with presystolic accentuation if the patient is in sinus rhythm. However, these signs are often modified by complicating factors including sclerosis and calcification of the cusps, a high pulmonary vascular resistance with consequent low blood flow, and other valvar defects. In addition a first loud heart sound may be palpable as a tapping impulse, and the murmur is often associated with a corresponding thrill.

In general, the longer the diastolic murmur the greater the severity of stenosis but there are exceptions and with a low cardiac output the murmur may become short or even disappear. In mild stenosis there may be only a short murmur. An apical systolic murmur is often present from an associated regurgitant jet or there may be a transmitted murmur here from aortic stenosis or tricuspid regurgitation.

If pulmonary hypertension is present there may be accentuation of the pulmonary component of the second sound and a right ventricular thrust from hypertrophy.

Right ventricular hypertrophy suggests dominant stenosis. Left ventricular hypertrophy, unless due to associated aortic valvar disease or systemic hypertension, suggests dominant regurgitation.

MITRAL REGURGITATION

The characteristic sign of mitral regurgitation is a long, harsh, apical systolic murmur which can be heard towards the left axilla and often as far as the left lung base. The murmur is long because of the pressure gradient throughout systole. If regurgitation is severe the first heart sound will be faint or absent and there will be a third heart sound early in diastole during the phase of rapid ventricular filling, and often also an early decrescendo, short, diastolic murmur due to increased blood flow from atrium to ventricle. In some forms of mitral regurgitation the systolic murmur occurs late in systole and rarely it is early or in midsystole.

MITRAL STENOSIS AND REGURGITATION

Rheumatic endocarditis often results in fusion and sclerosis of the cusps, which cannot come into apposition in systole, with the production of stenosis or regurgitation. In such cases the signs of these two valvar defects will be combined and often the practical problem arises as to the best form of surgical treatment.

The differentiation of dominant stenosis or regurgitation can often be made by consideration of all the clinical findings together with radiography and electrocardiography, but in cases of doubt cardiac catheterisation and left ventricular angiocardiography are necessary.

AORTIC STENOSIS

The characteristic sign of aortic stenosis is a harsh, systolic murmur which is audible over the upper sternum and to its left, and often down the left sternal border and at the apex. Occasionally it is loudest at the apex and may cause difficulty in differentiation from the murmur of mitral regurgitation or a transmitted murmur from elsewhere. Classically, the murmur is maximal in midsystole giving rise to a diamond shape on phonocardiography, but its precise configuration varies widely with the degree of obstruction and other factors. The murmur may be well heard over the carotid arteries but not necessarily so. There may or may not be an accompanying systolic thrill.

The aortic component of the second heart sound will be faint or absent, depending mainly on the mobility of the cusps.

Often, but by no means always, there is an accompanying systolic thrill. With significant obstruction, left ventricular hypertrophy will develop and, in due course, left ventricular failure. Reduced ventricular compliance from hypertrophy may be associated with an audible and palpable atrial sound and, with the onset of failure, the murmur becomes quieter and occasionally disappears to reappear after adequate treatment.

Characteristically the murmur has a different quality towards the apex, being of higher pitch and more musical. This fact is one source of confusion in differentiation from the murmur of mitral regurgitation which may of course also be present. The quality of maximum intensity in midsystole is retained.

The difficulty is increased if, as often happens, the heart sounds cannot be heard in the same situation as the murmur, so that precise timing is impossible. It is important to remember that an aortic systolic murmur of no haemodynamic significance is frequently present in the elderly and due to sclerosis of the cusps without a gradient across the valve. If severity of symptoms, or evidence of left ventricular hypertrophy, indicate that surgical treatment may be necessary, it is essential to be certain that obstruction to left ventricular outflow is at valvar level.

If an ejection sound is audible or if the valve is calcified there is no difficulty, but in the absence of these signs the alternative possibilities of sub- or occasionally supravalvar obstruction must be considered. Details of differential diagnosis are beyond the scope of this booklet but in the commonest variety of muscular subvalvar obstruction the principal signs are a quick rising pulse, a double impulse on palpation and a murmur which is loudest at the lower left sternal border.

AORTIC REGURGITATION

The characteristic sign of an aortic regurgitation is a diastolic murmur which begins with the second sound, continues throughout diastole and is of a blowing quality, maximal at the left sternal border.

With severe regurgitation and reduction of ventricular compliance from hypertrophy or left ventricular failure, the diastolic pressure will be raised and the murmur in consequence progressively abbreviated. Frequently there are signs also of aortic stenosis but aortic systolic murmur from the increased stroke output may be present without a gradient across the valve, especially if the cusps are abnormal.

The severity of stenosis may be indicated by peripheral signs such as exaggerated, carotid pulsation (Corrigan's sign), a collapsing (water hammer) radial pulse and muscle 'knock' and, of course, by left ventricular enlargement or hypertrophy. However, in the presence of associated aortic stenosis these peripheral signs may not be present although, at operation, the surgeon may consider that regurgitation is torrential (up to 5 litres per minute).

In the absence of corroborative signs it is not possible to differentiate an early diastolic murmur at the left sternal border due to aortic regurgitation from one due to pulmonary regurgitation by auscultation alone.

Aortic regurgitation, like aortic stenosis, is a matter of degree and in clinical practice the whole spectrum of severity is found.

Mild aortic regurgitation is probably the most benign of all acquired valvar defects because the left ventricle is well able to compensate for the increase in stroke volume for a life of normal span. However, there is always the risk of infective endocarditis.

When resulting from rheumatic fever the mitral valve is usually, but not always, also affected.

TRICUSPID DISEASE

Auscultatory signs of tricuspid disease are often overlooked. This is partly because its presence is not specifically considered in every patient with rheumatic heart disease but also because in most cases there are in addition murmurs from mitral and aortic valvar disease.

Diagnosis is facilitated by initial observation of the jugular venous pulse. Most patients with severe tricuspid stenosis maintain sinus rhythm and an exaggerated and characteristically flicking presystolic wave from atrial systole may be observed, particularly if the patient is reclining at only a few degrees from the horizontal. Initial detection of this sign should lead to the correct interpretation of the presystolic murmur. This murmur is often exceptionally clear, appears to originate close under the stethoscope and increases on inspiration.

The mid-diastolic murmur of tricuspid stenosis is usually best heard between the sternum and the apex, does not have the characteristic, rumbling quality of that due to mitral stenosis and, by contrast, it increases with inspiration.

These murmurs will be most readily detected if the patient is first instructed how best to breathe for their elicitation—by taking a slow, deep breath and then holding it in full inspiration whilst auscultation continues. The process is then reversed. In this way the characteristic waxing and waning will be most evident.

Likewise, in tricuspid regurgitation a systolic murmur is often audible in the same region and increases or only becomes audible during deep inspiration. However, if the right atrial (ventricular filling pressure) is high there may be no changes on respiration.

If there is right sided cardiac enlargement with clockwise rotation, as viewed from the apex, the murmur will be loudest at the apex. Occasionally, with extreme mitral stenosis and low blood flow the tricuspid systolic murmur may be the *only* auscultatory sign in a patient with severe mitral stenosis.

In tricuspid regurgitation there will be a systolic wave in the jugular venous pulse but often only in the deep vessels which can be indirectly observed, and systolic pulsation of the liver.

Tricuspid regurgitation may result with right ventricular failure from any cause.

COARCTATION OF THE AORTA

The systolic murmur originating at the site of obstruction in the descending aorta is loudest over the spine but usually also audible anteriorly.

There may also be a systolic murmur from a frequently associated, malformed aortic valve, from calcareous stenosis in such a valve, and sometimes from dilated collateral vessels. With complete occlusion of the aorta there will be no murmur from the area of coarctation but usually loud systolic murmurs from collateral vessels.

With severe narrowing but incomplete obstruction there may

be a continuous murmur over the spine and anteriorly the diastolic component may be mistaken for aortic regurgitation.

An aortic diastolic murmur may be present from congenital malformation of the valve or to dilatation of the valve ring secondary to the systemic hypertension. Rarely an apical diastolic murmur is present and probably due to relative mitral stenosis from dilatation of the left ventricle.

PATENT DUCTUS ARTERIOSUS

The characteristic sign is a continuous murmur which is maximal in late systole and loudest at the upper left sternal border or a little further out. There may or may not be an accompanying thrill.

With a large run-off from aorta to pulmonary artery there may be a somewhat collapsing pulse, an apical diastolic murmur from the increased blood flow across the mitral valve and a prominent left ventricular impulse.

PULMONARY STENOSIS

The characteristic signs are a harsh systolic murmur and thrill at the upper left sternal border together with an ejection click. With severe stenosis there will be a right ventricular thrust and often an exaggerated *a* wave in the jugular venous pulse and a presystolic triple rhythm.

Pulmonary stenosis may be associated with a left-to-right shunt at atrial or ventricular levels.

Sometimes the obstruction to right ventricular outflow is at subvalvar level involving the infundibulum of the right ventricle.

ATRIAL SEPTAL DEFECT

The characteristic signs are audible splitting of the second heart sound in expiration with fixed splitting during inspiration, and a pulmonary systolic murmur.

With a large flow across the tricuspid valve there will be a corresponding murmur and right ventricular lift.

If there is a systolic murmur at the apex, an ostium primum defect with a cleft mitral valve should be suspected.

ANOMALOUS PULMONARY VENOUS DRAINAGE

When the pulmonary veins drain directly or indirectly into the right atrium, the physical signs are similar to those of an atrial septal defect.

VENTRICULAR SEPTAL DEFECT

The characteristic signs of a ventricular septal defect (VSD) are a pansystolic murmur and thrill maximal at the left sternal border. A thrill is not always present. When there is a large gradient across the defect the systolic murmur is long because it extends throughout the period in which pressure in the left ventricle exceeds that in the right. In most cases this would be throughout systole. In some, owing to obstruction to RV outflow at valvar or subvalvar level or from pulmonary hypertension, the murmur is abbreviated.

With a large shunt there will also be increased blood flow across the mitral valve and consequently a diastolic murmur at the apex.

A reversed (right-to-left) shunt does not itself cause a murmur but a systolic murmur is often present from associated obstruction to RV outflow.

The two components of the second heart sound may be abnormally but not very widely split. This may be due to shortening of LV systole, due to the double outlet, with early closure of the aortic valve and prolongation of RV systole from the increased stroke volume. If there is pulmonary hypertension the pulmonary component will be loud and splitting narrow.

FALLOT'S TETRALOGY

Fallot's tetralogy consists of a high ventricular septal defect, obstruction to right ventricular outflow at infundibular or valvar level, dextroposition of the aortic root which lies astride the septal defect, and right ventricular hypertrophy.

The characteristic signs are central cyanosis with clubbing of the fingers and polycythaemia, and a pulmonary systolic murmur. The right to left shunt does not itself produce a murmur. There is no right ventricular lift because of the double outlet to the right ventricle. The second sound is single from the aortic component which may be loud due to the anterior position of the aorta.

In contrast to isolated pulmonary stenosis there is no ejection click or presystolic triple rhythm.

NOTE ON OBSTRUCTION TO RIGHT VENTRICULAR OUTFLOW

The findings in valvar and subvalvar (infundibular) stenosis are different.

In valvar stenosis the pulmonary systolic murmur is accompanied by an ejection click, the click being due to the sudden arrest of the ascending stenosed dome of the malformed valve. In contrast to an aortic ejection click, the pulmonary click decreases on inspiration with corresponding increased clarity on expiration.

During inspiration venous return to the right side of the heart is increased with a rise in RV end-diastolic pressure and a decrease in pulmonary end-diastolic pressure due to the greater negativity of the intrapleural pressure. In consequence, the pulmonary valve is displaced upwards before it opens and with ventricular systole there is little further excursion and sudden arrest which is responsible for the click.

The student need not be concerned with these refinements which are mentioned only to illustrate the valvar or a combination of infundibular and valvar.

Blood flow across the septal defect is silent and the more severe the degree of obstruction to RV outflow the shorter the murmur. The aorta is large and somewhat anterior and usually there is a loud, clear, single second sound due to the aortic component.

In the extreme form of the tetralogy, known as pseudo truncus arteriosus on account of pulmonary atresia, there will be no pulmonary systolic murmur but often a continuous murmur due to blood flow through greatly dilated bronchial arteries.

CONGENITAL HEART DISEASE IN INFANCY

The diagnosis of congenital heart disease in infancy is often complex and difficult and requires special experience. This subject will not therefore be discussed in detail. However, it may be mentioned that surgical treatment can be carried out successfully at this age, for example for a patent ductus or coarctation of the aorta, or some palliative procedure to increase pulmonary blood flow. Consequently, referral to a special centre may be indicated soon after birth.

In childhood physical signs of congenital heart disease are very similar to those in adults.

REFERENCES

BRUNS, D. L. (1959) A general theory of the causes of murmurs in the cardiovascular system. *American Journal of Medicine*, **27,** 360.

LEATHAM, A. (1970) *Auscultation of the Heart and Phonocardiography.* London: Churchill.

LUISADA, A. (1965) *From Auscultation to Phonocardiography.* St Louis: Mosby.

MCKUSICK, V. (1958) *Cardiovascular Sound in Health and Disease.* Baltimore: Williams & Wilkins.

INDEX

a wave, 6, 7
A₂, 37
Age, 1
Aneurysm, dissecting, 89
Aneurysm, sinus of Valsalva, 91
Aneurysm, ventricular, 18, 104
Anaemia, 1, 2, 13
Angina, palpation in, 18
Annulus, dilatation of, 76
Anxiety and the circulation, 1, 6
Aortic regurgitation, 8, 10, 89, 90, 112
Aortic sclerosis, 70
Aortic stenosis, 8, 10, 69, 111
Apex beat, 17
Apical diastolic murmurs, 97
Apical systolic murmurs, 74
Arachnodactyly, 13
Arcus senilis, 2
Areas of auscultation, 30
Argyll Robertson pupils, 2
Arrhythmias (dysrhythmias), 107
Ascites, 20
Asystole, 103
Atrial component of first heart sound, 41
Atrial fibrillation, 7, 11, 109
Atrial flutter, 7, 11, 109
Atrial septal defect, 115
Atrial tachycardia, 7, 11, 109
Atrial triple rhythm (*see* Fourth heart sound)
Auscultation, 24
Auscultation, technique of, 26
Austin Flint murmur, 95, 97
AV dissociation, 39
AV fistula, 99

Basal systolic murmurs, 68
Bedside approach to tachycardia and dysrhythmias, 107
Bicuspid aortic valve, 70
Bisferiens pulse, 8
Biventricular hypertrophy, 18
Bradycardia, 11
Bruns theory, 33
Bundle branch block, left, 46
Bundle branch block, right, 45

c wave, 6
Cannon waves, 7
Capillary pulsation, 14
Cardiac compression, 106
Cardiac failure, 17
Cardiac enlargement, 18
Cardiac hypertrophy, 18
Cardiac impulse, 17
Cardiac impulse, tapping, 19
    thrusting, 18
Cardiac tamponade, 6, 107
Cardiomyopathy, 3, 77
Cardiorespiratory murmur, 84
Carey Coombs murmur, 97
Carotid artery, pulsation, 5, 8
Carotid artery, kinking, 9
Carotid pulse, 8
Carotid sinus, hypersensitivity, 9
Carotid sinus, pressure and massage, 9
Cheyne Stokes breathing, 2
Chordal rupture, 77
Clicks, systolic, 43, 44
Cirrhosis of liver, 20
Clubbing of fingers, 13
Coarctation of aorta, 8, 114
Collapsing pulse, 10, 113
Collateral vessels, 14
Congenital heart disease in infancy, 117
Constrictive pericarditis, 6, 58
Continuous murmurs, 99
Coronary AV fistula, 99
Corrigan's pulse, 8, 113
Cushing's syndrome, 1
Cyanosis, 2, 13

Depression of sternum, 1, 21
Dextrocardia, 17
Diastolic murmurs, 87
Displacement of heart, 17
Discipline of auscultation, 32
Down's syndrome, 1
Double impulse, 19
Drugs and auscultation, 30
Duroziez, 193
Dysfunction, papillary muscle, 76, 104
Ductus patent, 114
Dysrhythmias (arrhythmias), 107

Early diastolic murmurs, 89
Ejection click, 43
Ejection murmurs, 67, 69, 81
Embolism, pulmonary, 104
Embolism, systemic, 104
Endocarditis, infective, 2, 77
Epigastric pulsation, 20
Exercise and the heart, 30
Extracardiac sounds, 84
Extrasystoles, 108

Fallot's tetralogy, 116
Femoral pulse, 20
Fever, 2
First heart sound, 37, 39
Fixed splitting of second sound, 46
Flow murmurs, 70, 73, 97
Fourth heart sound, 19, 40, 55, 56
Friction, pericardial, 84
Functional murmurs, 76, 80

Gallop rhythm, 52, 57
Genesis of heart sounds and murmurs, 33
Gibson murmur, 99
Graham-Steell murmur, 91
Gout, 14
Gallavardin, 69

Haemic murmurs, 72, 81
Hands, examination of, 13
Heart block, 7
Hepatic pulsation, 20
Heart sounds, 32
Hyperpnoea, 2
Hypertension, pulmonary, 105
Hyperthyroidism, 11
Hypothyroidism, 1

Infancy, congenital heart disease in, 117
Idiopathic murmurs, 80
Innocent murmurs, 80
Intensity of heart sounds, 38, 39
Inspection of neck, 4
Inspection of abdomen, 20
Intracardiac phonocardiography, 34
Isolated murmurs, 80

Infective endocarditis, 1, 77
Irregular pulse, 11

Jaundice, 2
Jet, mitral regurgitant, 76
Jugular venous pressure, 5
Jugular venous pulse, 5–7
Jugular venous pressure and pulse, 5

Kinked carotid artery, 9
Knock, pericardial, 19
Kyphoscoliosis, 1, 21
Kussmaul's sign, 6

Late systolic murmur, 75
Left atrial systolic expansion, 18
Left-sided heart disease, 29, 56
Left ventricular hypertrophy, 18
Liver, cirrhosis of, 20
    pulsation of, 20
    palms, 14

Macroglossia, 3
Mammary souffle, 100
Marfan syndrome, 1, 23
Midsternal murmurs, 79
Midsystolic murmurs, 69
Mid-diastolic murmurs, 93
Mitral facies, 2
Mitral first sound, 93
Mitral diastolic murmurs, 93
Mitral regurgitation, 39
Mitral stenosis, 93
Mongolism (Down's syndrome), 1
Murmurs, 32, 63
    apical diastolic, 97
    aortic diastolic, 89
    Austin Flint, 95, 97
    aortic systolic, 68
    basal systolic, 68
    diastolic, 97
    cardiorespiratory, 4
    extracardiac, 84
    early, 89
    ejection, 67, 69, 81
    haemic, 72, 81
    late, 67
    mitral diastolic, 93
    mitral systolic, 75
    mitral regurgitant, 75

Murmurs,
  mitral stenosis, 93
  presystolic, 94
  parasternal, 78
  transmitted, 78
  vibratory, 80
  isolated systolic, 83
  pulmonary diastolic, 91
  pulmonary systolic, 71
  systolic, 67
  tricuspid diastolic, 113
  tricuspid systolic, 113
  tricuspid stenosis, 94
Myocardial infarction, acute, 102
  complications, 102
  triple rhythm, 103
Myocardiopathy, 3, 78
Myocardial failure, 55

Neck, inspection and palpation of, 5
Neuromuscular disorders, 22
Nodules, rheumatic, 14
  rheumatoid, 14

Obesity, 1
Observation, 1
Obstruction to left ventricular outflow, 70
Obstruction to right ventricular outflow, 117
Opening snap of mitral valve, 58, 60
Osler's nodes, 14

Palpation of anterior chest wall, 17
Pansystolic murmurs, 82
Papillary muscle, dysfunction, 76, 104
  rupture, 76
Paradoxical (reversed) splitting, 46
Parasternal murmurs, 78
Patent ductus arteriosus, 115
Pathological triple rhythm, 55, 56, 60
Pericardial constriction, 6, 58
Pericardial effusion, 11, 106
Pericardial friction, 84
Pericardial knock, 19, 60
Pericardial rub, 84
Pericarditis in myocardial infarction, 104
Pericarditis, constrictive, 6, 11, 58
Petechiae, 2
Phonocardiography, 34
Physiological triple rhythm, 54, 56
'Pistol shot', 90
Posture and auscultation, 28
Pregnancy, 1
Presystolic murmurs, 42, 94

Pulmonary arteriovenous fistulae, 100
Pulmonary artery, dilatation of, 73
Pulmonary embolism, 104
Pulmonary hypertension, 105
Pulmonary stenosis, 72, 115
Pulmonary systolic murmur, 71
Pulmonary valve closure, 19
Pulmonary regurgitation, 91
Pulmonary blood flow, 72
Pulse, carotid, 8
  radial, 10
Pulsus paradoxus, 11
Pulsus alternans, 11

Qualities of heart sounds, 38

Radial pulse, 10
Regurgitant murmurs, 82
Regurgitant jet in mitral stenosis, 76
Respiratory variations, heart murmurs, 28
  heart sounds, 28
  pulse, 11
  venous pulsations, 5, 6
Reversed (paradoxical) splitting, 46
Rheumatoid arthritis, 3
Rheumatic nodules, 14
Rheumatoid nodules, 14
Right-sided heart disease, 29, 57
Ruptured chordae, 77
Ruptured mitral cusp, 78
Ruptured papillary muscle, 77

s wave, 6
S_2, 44
Scleroderma (systemic sclerosis), 3, 14
Sclerosis, aortic valve, 70
Scoliosis, 21
Single second sound, 47
Shock, 163
Skeletal deformities, 11
Snap, opening, 58
Sounds, heart, 32, 33
Splinter haemorrhages, 13
Splenic enlargement, 30
Splitting of first sound, 21
Splitting of second sound, 44, 46
Spondylosis, 21
Splitting paradoxical, 46
Sternal depression, 21
Sternal lift, 18
Stethoscope, 25
Straight-back syndrome, 22
Subvalvar obstruction, 70, 72
Sudden death in myocardial infarction, 103

Summation gallop, 58
Supraclavicular murmur, 70
Systemic sclerosis (scleroderma), 3
Supravalvar obstruction, 70
Systolic expansion of left atrium, 18
Systolic clicks, 43, 44
Systolic murmurs, 67, 68, 71, 75
Systolic pulsations, abnormal, 18

Tachycardia, 11
    bedside approach to, 107
Tamponade, cardiac, 107
Tapping impulse, 19
Third heart sound, 53–55
Thrills, 19
Third heart sound, 19, 53
Tongue, 3
Transmitted murmurs, 78
Traumatic mitral regurgitation, 78
Tricuspid regurgitation, 7, 79
Tricuspid stenosis, 94
Tricuspid disease, 113
Triple rhythm, 51

Unequal pulsations, 55

v wave, 7
Valsalva manoeuvre, 30
Venous hum, 100
Venous pressure and pulse, 5
Ventricular filling sound, 54
Ventricular hypertrophy, 18
Ventricular septal defect, 116
Ventricular septum, rupture of, 104
Ventricular tachycardia, 110

Xanthelasma, 2
Xanthomata, 14
x descent, 7

y descent, 7